TABLE OF CONTENTS

INTERMITTENT FASTING

EASY KETO DIET

INTERMITTENT FASTING
A COMPLETE GUIDE TO WEIGHT LOSS AND CLEAN EATING

BY NATASHA BROWN

All information is intended only to help you cooperate with your doctor, in your efforts toward desirable weight levels and health. Only your doctor can determine what is right for you. In addition to regular check ups and medical supervision, from your doctor, before starting any other weight loss program, you should consult with your personal physician.

INTERMITTENT FASTING:
How Intermittent Fasting Can Launch You Onto The Road Of Weight Loss, Improved Health, Mental Acuity and Increased Longevity

Introduction

In the world of health, nutrition and weight loss, intermittent fasting has been getting quite a bit of press in the last few years. What you might not realize is that far from merely being the latest trend and brainchild of some celebrity personal trainer/nutritionist, intermittent fasting has been in existence for thousands of years! I have chosen to write this book for several reasons. First of all, I want to dispel some of the popular myths about intermittent fasting. Second, through the presentation of historical facts and the science behind fasting, I want to advocate for the efficacy of intermittent fasting. Finally, as someone who has incorporated intermittent fasting into their health regime, I want to expose you, the reader, to several variations of intermittent fasting, answer common questions people have about this health practice, offer you practical tips and tricks to get the most out of your intermittent fasting experience, help you avoid fasting mistakes and ultimately, give you the information and advice that will allow you to incorporate this health practice into your health regime as a positive life choice, that will empower you for the rest of your life!

Let's begin with the myth debunking...

- You need to eat often to burn calories. This is just not always true. I will get into the details of how your body processes a meal later in this book, but basically, many experts consider that you can't fool your body into speeding up its metabolism and burning more calories by eating more frequently.

- When you intermittently fast, your body thinks you're "starving" and shuts down. Again, not true. You can't trick your body into thinking it's starving by skipping meals or fasting for a finite amount of time.

- When you fast, you lose muscle. On the contrary. When you fast, you lose fat and may, over time, actually gain lean muscle.

- You should never skip breakfast. This particular myth may actually have two sources. The people we normally associate with skipping breakfast are often overweight people without a disciplined eating regime intermittent fasting requires a disciplined eating regime. Also, the marketers of breakfast foods; i.e., cereal manufacturers, have a BIG interest in keeping the breakfast myth alive.

- "Eat breakfast like a king, lunch like a queen and dinner like a pauper". We've all heard this one at some point in our dieting lives. The truth is that the time of day you eat something has no effect on how fast or slow you burn the calories. This can be easily proven by studies that have been conducted on people who fast because of religious reasons, and eat large amounts of food late at night after the sun has set.

- Fasting is just plain BAD for you. I end with this myth, because, ironically, by reading the rest of this book, you will find that not only is fasting NOT bad for your health, but it can profoundly improve your body by increasing insulin sensitivity and decreasing inflammation, improve your mind by boosting levels of beneficial brain hormones and improve your life, affecting genes that control protection against disease as well as longevity.

Intermittent Fasting is not a diet. It is a life choice. Diets ultimately don't work because once you finish the diet, and abandon the strict disciplines of said diet that allowed you to lose weight in the first place, unless you find a solid maintenance plan, you will regain the original weight you lost, and worse, may even add additional pounds. Intermittent Fasting can be used both to lose weight AND maintain weight loss. It is a discipline that will allow you to transition from an overweight state into a healthy weight state and will help you, as long as you choose to follow this discipline, to maintain and prolong a balanced, healthy lifestyle for the rest of your life. Viewed in this light, I believe intermittent fasting has the ability to inspire, motivate and sustain positive, healthful personal growth. Proof of the potential physical, mental and spiritual benefits of intermittent fasting can be found throughout history, in the health regimes of countless elite athletes, living and competing in the present day and innumerable scientific studies being conducted to advance the quality of life for future generations.

If I haven't yet managed to convince you to read further, there is one more reason to consider embracing the lifestyle choice of intermittent fasting. Unlike diets, intermittent fasting doesn't ban certain foods. Sustained positive choice always requires balance. In the case of intermittent fasting, this balance is centered between indulgence and disciplined restraint. There will always be food-centered holidays and celebrations, and with the mindful planning and discipline that intermittent fasting entails, these occasions can be experienced fully without guilt or shame, with the supportive knowledge that tomorrow is truly another day that can balance the excesses of the past with a sensible, healthy, reliable intermittent fasting regime. It is only when you "celebrate" with food every day, that the balance is tipped and weight gain and other systemic health problems are given the opportunity to emerge.

Please note: Everyone's individual health base line is different and may require customized adaptations to a generic lifestyle choice. I urge you to share your plans to add intermittent fasting into your health regime with a medical professional before starting any type of program, to ensure you are proceeding in the most healthful and beneficial way for your individual health concerns.

The History of Fasting

This section has been included to conclusively prove that fasting has been around as long as civilization, and as a matter of fact, arguably even before, as can be witnessed by your pet dog or cat's fasting behavior when they have eaten something that doesn't agree with them or suffered some other illness. For the purposes of this book, I am focusing on the history of fasting as it pertains to religious, spiritual and medical usage.

Let's start with religious fasting. Excepting Zoroastrianism, a religion founded by a Persian prophet that forbids fasting (but does avoid eating meat four days a month!), one can hardly name a religion that does not historically include fasting in its observances in one fashion or another, for a wide spectrum of reasons.

Normally, the go-to source for religious fasting is the period of Ramadan, an approximately month-long period of time observed by Muslims around the world. During this period, eating and drinking is abstained from during daylight hours. The fast is then broken after sunset, usually by a large meal. Fasting is observed during Ramadan as an act of abstinence, as they strive to cleanse both body and soul and increase taqwa, or good deeds.

Muslims have always believed that by reducing overindulgence in food and eating only enough to quell hunger pangs, as well as maintaining normal daily physical activity during Ramadan, they are viscerally reaffirming their religious goals of always striving to attain virtuous behavior, character and habits in thought and deed. Christianity also has a long rich history of fasting, most notably during the Lenten period when fasting is also required by Roman Catholics as an act of abstinence and to represent and reenact the 40 days and nights Jesus spent alone, fasting in the wilderness.

In Judaism, fasting requires complete abstinence from food and drink, including water, and occurs on 6 days of the year, most notably Yom Kippur, which is considered the most important day of the Jewish year. Fasting on Yom Kippur represents atonement and repentance for all one's sins and transgressions from the past year.

Many Buddhist monks and nuns follow Vinaya rules and rarely eat after each day's noon meal. They do not consider this a fast, but more a part of their disciplined regimen, which they believe, helps them in meditation and general good health.

As I mentioned at the beginning of this chapter, there are many lesser known fasting traditions and rituals associated with religion and spirituality around the world. Here is just a sampling of a few of them:

- Eastern Orthodoxy: Fasting is tied to the principle between the body (Soma) and the soul (Pnevma). Orthodox Christians regard body and soul as a single unity and believe that what happens to one has an effect on the other (known as the Psychosomatic Union). Fasting takes up much of the

Eastern Orthodox calendar and is not enacted to suffer, but rather to guard against gluttony as well as negative thoughts, words and deeds. The fasting is always accompanied by prayer and almsgiving, or donations to charity or individuals in need.

- Church of the East: All Christians of Syriac traditions have practiced a pre-Lenten fasting event called the Nineveh Fast since the 6th century! During that time, a plague afflicted this region, which we now know as modern-day Iraq. Out of fear and desperation the people ran to their Bishop for a solution. The Bishop referred to scripture and ordered a three-day fast to ask God for forgiveness, based upon the story of Jonah in the Old Testament. Legend has it that after the three days the plague disappeared.

- Mormons: Members of the Mormon Church are encouraged to fast the first Sunday of each month. During these "Fast Sundays" they skip two meals for a total of 24 hours. Any money they save by not purchasing or preparing these two meals is donated to the church, which, in turn uses the money to help the needy.

- Hinduism: Fasting takes on many forms and variations in the Hindu religion, based on personal beliefs and local custom. Certain days of the week are designated for one's personal creed as well as favorite deities. Thursdays, for example, are a common fasting day for Hindus of northern India, who wear yellow clothing and worship Vrhaspati Mahadeva or Guru.

- Yoga: Practitioners of the yoga principle believe a fast should be maintained on the Full Moon day of each month, and to spend the entire day with a positive spiritual attitude

- Taoism: Fasting practices originated as a Daoist technique for becoming immortal and later became a traditional Chinese medical cure for Sanshi, or the "Three corpses", life-shortening spirits thought to reside in the human body.

- Sikhism: Sikhs only believe in fasting for medical reasons and when fasting for health are encouraged to remember to act with honesty, sincerity and to control desires.

Interestingly, no matter the form, intensity, length or reasoning for fasting in these religions and spiritual groups, all recommend cautions to individuals who are in some way not capable physically of the rigors of abstaining from nutrition. These include: children, the elderly, those who are medically fragile, pregnant, nursing

are constantly in the process of digestion and elimination.

If we begin to incorporate intermittent fasting into our eating regime, we begin to SCHEDULE periods of time of longer than 6 hours (when we aren't asleep) and allow our bodies the opportunity to experience entering the FASTING state more frequently.

What happens when our bodies are in the FASTING State?

- We burn through our normal energy stores of sugar, or GLUCOSE
- We find alternate sources of energy to burn in our body, including old protein, consisting of connective tissue, skin, old cells and other deitrus, which needs to be eliminated as well as...FAT!

If we were to stop right here, I think it's pretty obvious we could easily conclude that fasting helps our bodies not only burn energy sources more efficiently, but also repurposes fat and other undesirable elements in our body as alternative energy sources. In this way, not only are we thoroughly using up ALL energy resources, good and bad, but also, we are detoxing our bodies of old, used up material at the same time!

Here are a few more things that happen when our bodies are in a FASTING State:

- Leptin and Ghrelin Levels– Leptin and Ghrelin are basically the "appetite" hormones. Leptin tells your body to store fat and sends you hunger signals. Ghrelin tells your brain that your body is hungry. When your body is in a FASTING State it allows the panic buttons of Leptin and Ghrelin to be RESET! Thus, these two alarmist hormones settle down and stop being the "little boys who cried HUNGRY" all the time.

- Autophagy – This is a fancy word for the deep-cleaning process that our miraculous bodies attempt to do on top of everything else 24/7. Eating and Digestion get in the way of this process. However, when a body is in FASTING State, the digestive system gets a well-deserved break and clears the path for Autophagy to occur. Between our fasting bodies burning up fat stores and old used up bodily materials and focused periods of Autophagy, fasting enables our bodies to experience a good old-fashioned Autumn Leaf Fire and a thorough Spring Cleaning in one fell swoop!

These are just a few of the endlessly fascinating things that happen in our bodies when they are experiencing a FASTING State. If you, like me are a lifelong student -- the continued study of intermittent fasting will open up the door to endless learning opportunities. The more we understand how our bodies operate, as well as how best to maintain them, the more they will thank and reward us throughout our lifetime.

The Benefits of Intermittent Fasting

I think already, it is becoming quite obvious that Intermittent Fasting can be an effective and beneficial lifestyle choice for people looking to recover and/or maintain their health. While I tried to focus only on the history and science of fasting in the first two chapters, it became increasingly difficult to explore these two elements of intermittent fasting without touting at least a few of the benefits – as a form of spiritual communication, as an alternative health therapy throughout history and as a caloric regulator and physiological detoxifier.

In this chapter, I want to expand upon the list of the potential benefits of intermittent fasting and include as many lenses as possible through which to view the opportunities and rewards of this popular and effective health and wellness regime.

Physical Benefits

- Weight loss – intermittent fasting, when paired with clean, organic nutritious food eaten in moderation and the added bonus of physical activity, can result in steady, consistent weight loss that stays off!

- Targeted Belly Fat Loss – this harmful abdominal cavity fat can deposit around your internal organs and release proteins and hormones, which causes inflammation and may affect how well you break down sugars and fats. Intermittent fasting is the ideal solution for this stubborn weight gain, when paired with sugar reduction, increased healthy fats, sleep and stress reduction.

- Maintenance and potential gain of lean muscle mass – Many weight trainers and other elite athletes swear by intermittent fasting when training to help them maintain lean muscle mass and decrease total body fat.

Mental Benefits

- Improved metabolism, which is beneficial to Brain Health, Metabolism is the name for the crucial chemical reactions that happen in your cells. We talk about having a fast or slow metabolism all the time, without really understanding how vital it is to conversion of food to fuel, composing the building blocks for proteins and carbohydrates and the elimination of cellular waste.
- Improved Ketone production. Ketone is a chemical that protects the brain when there is a decrease of available glucose.
- May reduce symptoms of depression by regulating insulin and blood sugar levels.
- Enhances performance on memory tests in the elderly
- May play preventative role in those suffering from anxiety through regulation

of glucose and decreased oxidative stress. Oxidative stress happens when the body can't detox the harmful effects of free radicals (uncharged molecules) fast enough.

Systemic Benefits

- Cellular Repair – through autophagy, which is given more focus in a FASTING State.
- Hormonal Rebalancing – Insulin Levels and Insulin Resistance; Leptin; Ghrelin Also, Human Growth Hormone increases and facilitates fat burning and muscle gain
- Gene protection – Related to longevity and protection against diseases, including promising research on cancer
- Reduces Oxidative stress, damage and inflammation in the body

Quality of Life Benefits

- May improve sleep patterns – If your intermittent fasting schedule includes eating a meal 3 to 4 hours before sleeping, and includes carbohydrates, your sleep quality and quantity could improve due to increased production of serotonin, a chemical in the body that helps regulate cyclic body processes, such as the sleep cycle, as well as contributing to feelings of happiness and wellbeing.

- Increased stamina – Athletes who exercise on an empty stomach have experienced more energy and stamina. It is believed that the combination of fasting and exercising triggers internal catalysts that force the breakdown of sugars and fat into energy, without sacrificing muscle mass.

Behavioral Benefits

- Improves appetite control – Intermittent Fasting allows you to discern between mental and physical hunger
- Helps with food cravings – As your Leptin and Ghrelin levels reset to your intermittent fasting schedule, old triggers to eat certain foods at certain times will be erased. Also, intermittent fasting doesn't ban certain foods; only the time period in which you can consume them!
- Develops an appreciation for high quality food—when you learn to eat within a certain time frame, and fast through another, you learn to appreciate the gift of eating good quality food. You may notice that you savor food more, eating it more slowly, and that you have a much keener sense of when you are becoming full. You will also discover certain, high quality food

sources such as whey protein, green vegetables and berries are ingested and incorporated faster into your system, due to their nutritionally dense makeup.

Fiscal and Time-Saving Benefits

- Save money – Depending on your intermittent fasting schedule, you could end up skipping 7 meals or more a week. As long as you don't add the caloric totals of these meals to the meals you DO consume during intermittent fasting, you are basically cutting at least a day's worth of food out of your budget. Take a page from the Mormon faith and add up how much money you save by not purchasing and preparing these meals. Whether you pay that savings forward or save it for a rainy day is up to you!

- Save time – This particular benefit personally resonates with me. As a former dieter, I can say with the voice of an expert, that many of the miracle diets and fads I tried, in my quest to lose weight, not only included lots of really expensive ingredients in little quantities that resulted in even more waste, but the elaborate preparation required of these meals, took hours away from my life that I would never get back. When you choose to fast intermittently, you automatically save a certain percentage of weekly food prep basically because you SKIP the entire process. It's up to you how plain or fancy your remaining meals are. The important thing is to eat a balanced, clean, organic nutritious menu of food. And if you overindulge a day or two on vacation? Tomorrow is truly another day.

Personal Growth Benefits

- Taking a on a physical and mental challenge and being rewarded with the ability to balance health and nutritional needs.
- Acquiring a great tool for strength training or other athletic challenges.
- Experiencing consistent balanced control over important life choices.
- Gaining the flexibility and freedom to choose when you eat socially with friends and family, and when you take a planned break.
- Experiencing Mind/Body connection in a visceral manner that regulates when, why and how you eat.
- Learning how to be mindful when eating
- Experiencing delayed gratification rather than immediate gratification
- Developing resilience in a controlled setting

- Learning how to respect boundaries and how to be nutritionally creative within them

As I hope you can see by the diverse spectrum of benefits I've included above, I personally believe that the practice of Intermittent Fasting offers you much, much more than a diet. As I've stated before, it's an important, valuable life choice – the rewards that will be gained from incorporating it into your health regime can easily be scaffolded into many other parts of your life. I am a big advocate of connecting mind, body and spirit into a cohesive, healthy, balanced whole, transforming us all into empowered individuals; ready to take on all the opportunities this world has to offer!

Three Major Types of Intermittent Fasting

Intermittent Fasting, as we know it today, has been in existence roughly since the turn of the millennium. In the past seventeen years, it has gained more and more traction, as more research is conducted, more health, nutrition and athletic groups have incorporated it into their programs and more and more people have adopted it as a viable, sustainable life choice. When you think about it, almost two decades is an impressive run for something that was initially dismissed by many as an unhealthy fad! There are probably as many variations of intermittent fasting on the market today as there are health and wellness sites, so in order to expose you to as wide a selection of available plans within the confines of this book, I have chosen to focus on three major types: Whole Day Fasting (WDF); 5:2 Intermittent Fasting; and Timed Restricted Fasting (TRF).

Whole Day Fasting (WDF)

Whole Day Fasting was developed and made popular by Brad Pilon, who wrote the book, *Eat Stop Eat*. The basic concept of this intermittent fasting plan is to fast for 24 hours once or twice a week. During the fasting period, no food is consumed but calorie-free beverages are freely permitted (and encouraged). A typical fast day might start after your evening meal, at 7 pm on a Tuesday. You then would fast from all food until 7 pm on Wednesday, at which time you would go back to normal eating. For the next couple of days, you would eat normally (about 2000 calories for women; 2500 for men) and then you would have another 24 hour fast and repeat the schedule. The main rule would be NEVER to fast for two days in a row, or fast more than two times in one week. Maintenance of whole day fasting like this would result in cutting 2/7 of your normal weekly food consumption.

Optimally, your caloric goal on fast days would be as little as possible, drinking tea, coffee, plain or sparkling water and other zero-calorie beverages. The key to non-fasting days would be moderation and balance, as overeating on these days could start to undo what you accomplished during the fast. This is especially important if you are intermittently fasting with the primary goal of losing weight. However, you do not have to avoid any specific foods, although lots of fruits, vegetables and spices are recommended.

Pilon specifically developed this particular intermittent fasting plan as part of a fitness regime that included resistance and weight training to maintain and build lean muscle, rather than cardio-based routines, which might be too taxing, especially on fasting days. The recommended training schedule would be 3 to 4 times a week.

5:2 Intermittent Fasting

5:2 fasting, also known as The Fast Diet, was popularized by Michael Mosley, a British doctor. Like Whole Day Fasting, participants eat normally 5 days of the week, but instead of a complete fast on the other 2 days, restrict calories to 500-600 a day. This eating pattern depends more on timing than food choice and only requires counting calories two days a week, but is obviously, not as restrictive as the 24 hour fasting periods of Whole Day Fasting. Many who choose this form of intermittent fasting, designate Mondays and Thursdays as the two days they reduce caloric intake to between 500 (for women) and 600 (for men) calories. Whichever days you choose, the one rule is to have at least ONE non-fasting day between the two fasting days.

Mosely recommends eating 3 small or 2 slightly bigger meals a day on the 2 fasting days, and to focus on high fiber, high protein foods that will help you feel full without extra calorie consumption. Your total caloric consumption on fast days should equal 25% of your normal daily food consumption. Therefore, in one week you would theoretically be cutting out 75% of your calories on 2 out of 7 days, IF you don't go over 2000 (women) or 2400 (men) calories a day on the remaining 5 days.

The 5:2 plan also advocates exercise, and basically says, with medical clearance, that after the initial transition weeks, ANY exercise regime that is normally followed can be continued through fast days, although again, intense cardio is not specifically advocated.

The 5:2 plan also takes BMI (Body Mass Index), BMR (Basal Metabolic Rate) and TDEE (Total Daily Energy Expenditure) into account. BMI calculates how much body fat you have, in proportion to your height and weight. BMI measures the amount of calories you would burn if you just sat and did nothing for a 24-hour period. TDEE equals the number of calories you consume in a day when your BMR is scaled to a level of activity. In other words, how many calories a day you need to maintain your current weight, and depending upon how active you are, how many calories a day you should consume on the 5 days you aren't fasting.

Although this gets a bit technical and may seem to fly in the face of the principle that intermittent fasting is great because you don't need to worry about what you eat on non-fasting days, it's really just a more complicated way to remember moderation, especially if your goal is to lose weight.

Timed Restricted Fasting (TRF)

Time Restricted Fasting also known as Leangains, was developed and popularized by Martin Berkhan, a professional fitness writer and consultant, who revolutionized the fitness scene when he proposed that intermittent fasting was better for athletes in training (specifically body builders) than eating small meals every 2 to 3 hours. The basic concept of Timed Restricted Fasting is to fast for 16 hours a day and then eat in the remaining 8-hour window of time. There are no food restrictions during the 8-hour feeding period, as long as you meet your daily caloric and macronutrient target. What are macronutrients? Macronutrients (or macros) are a fancy term for the types of food needed by a living organism. For humans this means carbohydrates, fats and proteins, which are the three basic components of every diet! Getting the proportions of these three nutrients right makes a big difference, when trying to maintain or lose weight. Some people claim that counting macros is much more effective than counting calories when controlling weight. For the purposes of understanding macros to calories the following explains what each macro counts as, in caloric terms:

- Protein – equal to 4 calories per gram
- Carbohydrates –equal to 4 calories per gram
- Fats – equal to 9 calories per gram

Once you have this formula down, you can determine your personal macronutrient targets. A common split is 40/40/20. In other words, 40% of your calories should be spent on protein, 40% on carbohydrates and 20% on fats. Again, compared to the simplicity of Whole Day Fasting, all of this may seem complicated and defeat the purpose of intermittent fasting, but it really comes down to your personal goals and what level of nutrition and fitness comprehension resonates with you. It can be as simple as moderation or as complex as formulating your daily macronutrient needs – and it means the same thing!

Time Restricted Fasting was specifically designed to be used by body builders who were basically tired of eating constantly like frenzied birds; feeling "half-starved" all of the time and wanted to be able to eat large meals some of the time with relative freedom. It was also designed as a response to athletes who were tired of having to miss many social events, as the timing and food-themed tones of most of them didn't fit into their 2-3 hour mini-meal schedule.

It goes without saying that Time Restricted Fasting advocates for the addition of physical activity, as intense training and intermittent fasting go hand in hand in this particular version. Again, cardio activities take a back seat to resistance and weight training in this scenario.

The three types of Intermittent Fasting I have chosen to highlight in this section are currently among the most popular and trending today, but are certainly NOT the only ways in which you can experience intermittent fasting. Other variations include: *The Warrior Diet*, a 20-hour fasting sequence with one meal a day, written by Ori Hofmekler, *The UpDayDownDay Diet*, written by Dr. James Johnson, which uses an alternative day intermittent fasting approach and focuses on targeting what he refers to as the "skinny" gene, and *Fat Loss Forever*, a hybrid of *Eat Stop Eat*, *Warrior Diet* and *Leangains*, that features a cheat day followed by a 36 hour fast, started by John Romaniello and Dan Go.

Alternatively, once you have a basic understanding of the basic principles of intermittent fasting and have figured out your own goals, there is no reason why you can't pick up your favorite "best practices" from these variations, and devise a customized intermittent fasting program that meets your own needs! I've written the following chapters of this book with the intention of helping you implement the tools of intermittent fasting into your daily life, whether your goals include weight loss, weight maintenance, nutritional improvement and consistency, physical training goals, increased stamina and endurance, appetite control or any of the other numerous nutrition/health and wellness issues that may be interfering with the balance of your daily life. Let's get started!

Intermittent Fasting For Weight Loss And The "Magic Bullet" Of Exercise

If one of your health goals for using intermittent fasting is weight loss, it's important to establish some base lines before starting your journey. First of all, you need to figure out how many calories you need in order to facilitate a healthy weight loss, keeping in mind, that the addition of ANY kind of intermittent fasting practice will automatically eliminate a percentage of calories per time period fasted X how many meals you skip. As I mentioned earlier, then recommended daily calorie intake for maintaining healthy body weight is 2000 for women and 2500 for men. It is also commonly accepted that cutting back 500 calories a day, to 1500 for women and 2000 for men, will optimize weight loss of up to one pound per week.

However, this is only a standard. Everyone is different, and medical needs, stage of life needs, activity levels, etc. should always be factored in. Medical clearance for any sort of weight reduction is recommended, should be sought out as an important source of advice and/or feedback during the weight loss process.

Please don't be disappointed that I am talking about calories and restriction. I know you've probably been excited about intermittent fasting because one if it's most attractive selling points is the "eat all you want" aspect on non-fasting days. If you don't want to lose more than a couple of pounds or are looking to accomplish other health/nutrition goals, this benefit holds fast, albeit, perhaps it should be edited to read "Eat all the clean organic, nutrient dense food you want", or "eat all the macronutrients that will contribute to your lean muscle mass". OKAY... maybe these variations don't exactly say, "Gorge to your heart's content", but compared to many calorie restrictive diets.... It's a good thing!

And speaking of calorie restrictive DIETS...don't you think using the tool of intermittent periods of fasting, interspersed with "normal" periods of moderation sound a heck of a lot better than eating cabbage soup three times a day or prepping 6 mini meals every night before you head to bed? I thought so! Also, when I think of intermittent fasting I think of endless opportunities to get the whole weight loss battle right – if, God forbid, you have an occasional overindulgent non-fasting day all you need to do to reset is go to sleep, unrepentant because tomorrow or the next day offers the opportunity to redeem yourself with a period of fasting. Try that in week two or three of some draconian food-deprived diet and chances are you'll be slipping off that wagon faster than that piece of cake you devoured at your friend's birthday party!

But I digress...If you aren't satisfied with a minimum standard of how many calories you should be consuming per day, including intermittent fasting there is a formula to customize this number for your personal needs. Borrowing from 5:2 intermittent fasting and The Fast Diet, here's how to figure out your TDEE (Total Daily Energy Expenditure):

Note: This formula uses the metric system. 1 kg = 2.2 pounds; 1 inch = 2.54 cm

FIRST: Calculate your BMR (Basal Metabolic Rate)

Women: BMR = 655 + (9.6 X weight in kg) + (1.8 X height in cm) – (4.7 x age in years)

Men: BMR = 66 + (13.7 X weight in kg) + (5 X height in cm) – (6.8 X age in years)

Multiply the number in parenthesis first, then you can add and subtract

EX: Female
Age 55 years
Weight: 197 lbs. (89.54 kg)
Height: 5' 4" (162.56 cm)
655 + (9.6 X433.4 kg) + (1.8 X 162.56 cm) – (4.7 X 55) = 1,549 calories/day (rounded up)

SECOND: Calculate TDEE
TDEE = BMR X Activity Factor

Activity Factor:
Sedentary (little or no exercise) = 1.2

Lightly Active (light exercise 1-3 days/week) = 1.375

Moderately Active (exercise 3-5 days/week) = 1.55

Heavy Exercise (exercise 6-7 days/week) = 1.725

Very Heavy Exercise (physical labor; training 2X/day) = 1.9

EX: 1,549 calories X 1.375 (lightly active) = 2,129 calories a day needed to maintain current weight
In order for this woman to lose approximately 1 pound per week she would need to cut her daily calorie count by 500 calories, adjusting her TDEE to 1,629 calories a day.

WHEWWW! That wasn't easy! The good news is there are calculators and apps that will do all this work for you if math isn't among your strong suits. However, I always think it's worthwhile to understand how a rate is figured out and the bonus is the one thing that becomes abundantly clear when working out your TDEE is what a powerful tool physical activity can be in your weight loss journey.
How truthful were you when it came to figuring out your Activity Factor? Don't feel bad – most people overestimate how active they are. Were you surprised at how much you needed to move to be considered moderately active? The good news is physical activity; ANY physical activity can be added to your health regime, AT YOUR COMFORT LEVEL. I'm afraid we've all become accustomed to watching extreme weight loss reality shows and falling for the belief that in order to make a difference in weight loss, we need to immediately jump into the fray, overworking ourselves into a

dangerous, sweaty, sobbing mess in order to feel the burn.

FAIL! This is an extremely dangerous way to introduce exercise into your life and the chance of injury or emotional trauma is more than likely to ensure you will think 10 times before attempting to exercise again. Work out in this fashion and you will literally end up THE BIGGEST LOSER.

Instead, I offer you various physical activity options to try out at any level of the activity factor. Please read the following from beginning to end to see the possibilities and opportunities that await a human being currently at any level of fitness:

- Physical Activity Options for the Sedentary: Gentle yoga; chair yoga; walking with a friend; mall walking; tai chi; social dancing, i.e., folk, line, square; walking in a pool; gentle aqua aerobics; lawn games like croquet or bocce; light gardening or yard work. The key is to go at your own pace, stop whenever you need to and ignore people who try to push you beyond your limits. It's a lifelong process – not a race!

- Physical Activity for the Lightly Active: Start taking the stairs more often; park farther from your destination and walk the rest of the way; spring clean once a month; buy a pedometer or Fitbit and start keeping track of your steps; play with your kids or grandkids; go on family walks after dinner.

The key is to begin incorporating physical activity into your daily routine, while keeping up with the fun stuff you started when you were sedentary!

- Physical Activity for the Moderately Active: On days you don't have planned or scheduled physical activities, you should try to aim for 60 minutes of Lifestyle activity which could include house and garden work; biking or hiking with friends and family, swimming in your home pool or going to a lake or ocean beach for the afternoon and spending time swimming organized sports such as work softball or pickup basketball teams; volunteer physical labor for church or community as well as formal gym and swim classes; or scheduled jogging or biking sessions. The key at this point is to celebrate how far you've come from the couch and TV by honing your level of physical fitness in work and play.

- Physical Activity for the Heavy Exerciser: Challenge yourself with CrossFit; competitive sports such as tennis, swimming or ballroom dancing; mountain climbing and biking, cross country ski, long-distance hiking; train for and compete in marathons, and triathlons; cross-country biking vacations and races. Take the skills you've mastered in the gym and implement them in real-life activities. The key at this point is to discover and challenge your fitness at every opportunity. Learn new skills to keep the mind-body connection strong and keep advancing your personal best.

- Physical Activity for the Very Heavy Exerciser: Ironman events; elite tests of endurance such as Tough Guy UK; epic adventure races like Raid Gauloises or the Barkley 100 Trail Race; REI's Mount Kilimanjaro Climb; or elite mud runs like The Spartan Beast, which runs in various cities and dates. Remove any remaining limits and pit your skills against the best in the world! There's always room to grow and physically challenge yourself! Check out these events and more on the Internet. The World is your oyster!

The point of this is – that basically once you begin adding physical activity to your routine, there is literally no end point. Physical fitness at any age, level, ability or disability, knows no limit and is only made more achievable and exciting by the personal boundaries that we choose or that have been thrust upon us! Beginning a program of intermittent fasting is the perfect opportunity to discover the joys of physical fitness, while reaping the calorie burning, body freeing, flexibility and agility benefits that learning to move your body will offer you.

Twenty Questions About Intermittent Fasting!

The aim of this section is to answer any and all questions you might have at this point about intermittent fasting. I've tried to address questions related to fasting for weight loss as well as for people who are looking to maintain and/or otherwise amp up their health and wellness regime. If you have questions I didn't address, please send them in! I love getting feedback from my readers and using it to improve the books I write!

Which type of intermittent fasting should I choose to follow and why?

Many of the reasons for choosing one type of intermittent fasting over another will depend on personal preference, lifestyle as well as short and long-term goals. What I can do for you is list some advantages of each of the 3 types I described earlier in this book.

Whole Day Fasting

- o 1 to 2 days of fasting and 5 days of feeding give you greater flexibility when it comes to eating socially, or at home with family.
- o Works for those who resonate with "all or nothing" mentality
- o Fits in well with vacation and/or holiday plans

o   Allows for longer "recovery" time between fasting

o   Allows you to "get it all over with" in only 48 hours

5:2 Intermittent Fasting

o   The 2 minimal calorie days, still allow you to eat something

o   Feels less restrictive than Whole Day Fasting

o   Allows you to eat a bit after training session, even on "fast" days

o   Appeals to people who have issues about not eating at all for 24 hours

o   Might be a great way to introduce yourself or transition into intermittent fasting

Time Restricted Fasting

o   More attractive to people who resonate with a more consistent routine

o   The ability to fast and eat in one 24-hour period

o   The philosophy that every day is a brand-new opportunity to improve

o   Less chance of overindulging during feeding periods

o   Creates more structured boundaries

Please also remember, that there are many more

types, hybrids and versions of intermittent fasting available to choose from. The most important takeaway is that you find a plan that resonates with you! And if you can't find exactly the right fit for your needs, there's no reason you can't design your own plan. Finally, keeping in mind that ideally, intermittent fasting is a life-long choice, don't limit yourself to one way of fasting. Life changes, and when it does, it's important to be able to flex to new challenges. Fortunately, for us, there are a variety of ways to accomplish intermittent fasting!

How and what should I eat during feeding periods?

The short answer is: Any way and anything you want! The long answer needs to reflect what your nutrition goals are. If you are intermittently fasting to lose weight, you need to eat in moderation and make sure you don't "make up for lost time" in terms of the meals you skipped while fasting. No matter what type of fasting program you are following, it's important to know how many calories you should be aiming for a day, i.e., your TDEE minus 500 calories a day or more, depending on how much weight you would like to lose a week. But remember – if you are fasting, that 500 calories probably has already been saved! Isn't that great news!

If you are practicing intermittent fasting because you are a weight trainer and are sick of eating like a bird every 2 or 3 hours, then your feeding goals are going to be much different. You will need to make sure that you eat everything you missed during the fasting period, during the window of feeding time. Also, what you eat, i.e., how much protein vs how many carbs, will be important to continue to support your training. If you are training for a specific event such as a marathon or triathlon, you may need to up certain food groups, in preparation for the big day.

If you have decided to practice intermittent fasting in order to experience the many health and wellness benefits I listed previously, but you are satisfied with your current weight, you will need to be mindful that you are eating enough to satisfy your TDEE and that those food sources are as nutrient-dense, clean and organic as possible.

Choosing an intermittent fasting lifestyle can mean that an occasional indulgence will be balanced out by the majority of your healthy food choices. It really shouldn't mean that you fast intermittently so that you can binge on junk food and processed, GMO laden prepared foods. Intermittent Fasting is not a giant filter, magically cleansing you of your toxic food choices. It is a lifestyle that allows you to easily balance eating to live and living to eat.

I'm concerned…. Won't this mess up my circadian rhythms?

First of all, let's explain what circadian rhythms are! Basically, your circadian rhythm is your 24-hour internal clock that runs in the background of your consciousness and cycles your body between periods of sleep and wake. It's also known as your sleep/wake cycle. Typically, most adults experience the most profound dip in energy twice in a 24-hour cycle: once somewhere between 2 and 4 am, and once between 1 and 3 pm. These times can shift if you tend to be more nocturnal or a "morning" person. When you experience consistent, quality sleep you won't be as aware of these 2 cyclical decreases in energy.

If you are sleep deprived, you will. The lightness or darkness of your environment can trigger your circadian rhythms, as darkness cues your eyes to tell your brain that it's time to feel tired. Your brain then sends a signal to your body to release the hormone melatonin, which makes you physically tired. So, night and day as well as consistent sleep periods pretty much regulate your circadian rhythms.

Disruptions such as daylight savings time, travelling to another time zone, or watching late night TV can disrupt your circadian rhythms and you will pay for it the next day. Can intermittent fasting also disrupt circadian rhythms? The answer is interesting – it depends! The interesting part is that it is NOT because many intermittent fasting programs skip breakfast (although, as we have discussed several times, intermittent fasting and feeding times can be adjusted to personal preference). In actuality, our hunger is naturally at our lowest point upon waking, increases during the day, and peaks around 7 to 8 at night.

We in western civilization tend eat dinner around this time period because it conveniently coincides from when we get home from work and school commitments and reconvene as a family. Also, our internal levels of insulin are maximally stimulated at this time so eating dinner on the late side starts to feel like the perfect storm. When viewed in this light, no matter how you are eating (intermittently or at will) or what you are eating, doesn't matter as much as when you are eating. Perhaps, if instead we all took a page from the Mediterraneans, who eat their largest meal in the early afternoon, and then siesta it off with an afternoon nap, before returning to work and eating a light meal, later in the evening, we'd all benefit from our hormonal and circadian cycles working in perfect harmony! So bottom line: Intermittent fasting doesn't need to interrupt your circadian rhythm but waiting until 9 o'clock at night to catch up on the bulk of your eating could.

I think I need to take a break on weekends. Can I still do intermittent fasting?

If you choose to follow a daily intermittent fasting plan such as time restricted fasting, the answer is, sadly no – you would have to break the daily pattern to take a break on weekends. If, however you follow an intermittent fasting plan such as whole day intermittent fasting or 5: 2 intermittent fasting the answer to this question is a resounding YES!

In fact, as I believe I mentioned earlier, the recommended days for 5:2 fasting are Mondays and Thursdays, which when you think about it, couldn't work out better for taking the weekend off and indulging just a bit. Your fasting days basically "sandwich" (sorry about the pun!) the weekend, allowing you to eat much more freely, knowing you've just ended a fast and will enter another after the hopefully, minor excesses of the weekend!

I'm really concerned about losing muscle mass. How can I prevent this from happening while training and fasting intermittently?

As I've mentioned before, one of the benefits of using Intermittent Fasting methods while training or working out, is that you tend to lose FAT while maintaining lean muscle mass. But there are additional techniques you can employ to ensure that you will maintain, and if you choose, even gain lean muscle mass while intermittently fasting. Calorie and carbohydrate cycling are both great tools to add to your nutritional program. Cycle calories by eating more on the days you work out and less on your training days. In other words, add or decrease food intake during your feeding times, to coincide with training or rest days. This results in more energy to burn into muscle on training days and fewer calories to burn fat on your resting days.

If you follow this pattern consistently, you should end up having done both in one week. Carbohydrate cycle by increasing carb consumption on training days and decreasing carbs on resting days. The principle works the same way as caloric cycling. Finally, eat high protein all the time and decrease fat intake to moderate or low on resting days.

I'm not fasting to lose weight... How do I manage to eat enough food during my feeding window?

Okay, people who need to lose a few pounds – stop groaning and throwing things! This is just as much of a concern for people as counting calories is for others. When people incorporate intermittent fasting into their training schedule as an alternative to eating every two or three hours throughout the day, they gain time to eat socially with family and friends as well to eat normal sized plates of food, but there is also a transition challenge of eating enough calories when weight loss isn't a goal. Perhaps the easy answer would be to enjoy all that fattening ice-cream, cake and alcohol that most people can't – but we're talking about people who take their health and nutritional needs very seriously – at least most of the time. So, what are some nutrient-dense healthy choices that will add those extra needed calories?

- Nuts – great source of protein and fat and may protect you from heart attacks. Pine nuts pack the biggest caloric wallop at 673 calories for 3 ounces, but macadamias are no slouch either at 600 calories for 3 ounces.
- Peanuts and Peanut Butter – I know you already knew peanuts are NOT nuts. They are legumes and contain more than 30

essential nutrients and phytonutrients. They also contain Vitamin E, niacin, which helps lower cholesterol, and magnesium, which increases metabolism. 2 tablespoons of this miraculous stuff contains 7 grams of protein and 188 calories.

- Avocados – They're jam packed with antioxidants, vitamins, folate and potassium (60% more than bananas!). They're a great source of unsaturated fat and have been shown to reduce cholesterol when used to replace saturated fats like cheese. One avocado has 300 plus calories.
- Dried Fruit – Dried fruits contain more nutrients, greater fiber content and significantly greater phenol antioxidants as their fresh counterparts. Because it has been dried, its nutrients and calories are very concentrated. Dried fruits include apples, apricots, bananas, blueberries, cherries, grapes, mangos, papayas, peaches, pineapple, dates and figs. A small box of raisins has 129 calories, and cherries weigh in at 160 calories for a mere third of a cup!
- Olive Oil – 1 tablespoon of this golden, green goodness has 120 calories. Use it to cook, on salads, to dip whole grain bread in... This could be the ultimate condiment!
- Protein Shakes, smoothies, shakes and fresh squeezed juices – Celebrate your

need for extra calories and either hit up your local organic juice bar or make your own nutrient dense, calorie laden beverages! Just be sure the ingredients in the Protein Shakes contain high quality undenatured whey protein, that hasn't been exposed to high heat and had its amino acid cellular structure altered. And go light on even the natural sugars.

Fasting for all those hours seems overwhelming. What can I do to make it easier?

The first thing you can do to make intermittent fasting easier is to transition into it at your own pace. Start by fasting for as long as you feel comfortable and build up to the fasting program's recommended hours. If this feels like cheating, start with restricted time fasting, and if at first, even those hours of fasting feel overwhelming build up to their recommendations. This is a life choice; not a diet. Life choices take a lifetime to truly master. Here are some additional tips to help you on your intermittent fasting journey:

- Begin your fast after dinner – Eat your last meal around 7 pm. Go directly to Bed! Wake up at 7 am and BAM! 12 hours of your fast are already over. That's right! Sleep is the beginning faster's best friend!
- Drink Plenty of Water, Tea, Coffee, Sparkling Water, Cold Brewed Teas and

Coffees...Fill that empty stomach with hydrating zero calorie beverages. If you're not overly sensitive to caffeine, the coffee and teas will also give you a lift!

- Don't EVER fast more than two 24-hour periods in one week (this does not, of course count time restricted fasting, as you break that fast for 8 hours each day). Fasting up to two times a week basically cuts up to 30% of your calories. Fasting more than this cuts calories too much and may result in loss of energy and strength and could actually cause boomerang overeating!

How do I coordinate my training schedule to my intermittent fasting schedule?

If you use the fasting and feeding times of your intermittent fasting plan as the boundaries for your training sessions, you will end up with fasted training time that is followed by a replenishing main meal, provided you eat the appropriate foods that complement the workout you've just completed. Here's an example:

Noon: Do workout in fasted state

1 PM: Break 16- hour fast and consume 30 – 50% of daily calories by eating large meal with protein shake

7 PM: Eat balance of calories by eating large dinner

9PM – 1PM Next day: Fast for 16 hours

Please note: This is only an example. While it's important to follow a fasted workout with an ample, replenishing meal, the balance of the day's calories can be eaten at will, as long as the fasted state begins again at 9 pm

Is it ok to drink diet soda when I fast intermittently?

Ummm... Yessss... but why would you want to do that? Sorry about answering a question with a question – but it makes me pause to think that anyone – never mind a health-minded individual, still drinks diet soda. I don't mean to be blunt; but IT'S CHEMICALS, PEOPLE! There. I feel like I've done my duty. The other reason is, there is evidence-based proof that when you drink artificially sweetened beverages, you crave...SUGAR. Not a good thing, and I've got the generation of obese, type two diabetic children to prove it. There are so many great natural alternatives out there – If you need the bubbles, why not try sparkling water or seltzer in at least 50 different flavors – all still coming in at zero calories? Then there's cold brew packs of fruit and spice flavored teas and coffees – delicious as well as warming, soothing hot herbal and caffeinated teas. You can get organic "loaded" and decaf coffee, also in a variety of flavors and from coffee growers around the globe. It's probably the best time in history for zero calorie beverages.

Consider yourself a purist? Consider water – nature's eternal life source! And remember – you are only limited to zero calorie beverages during the fasted state. As you virtuously sip away you can plan ahead for all the delicious juices, lattes and smoothies that await you – in just a matter of hours!

Should I take vitamins when I intermittently fast?

It is more important than ever to take vitamins and supplements when fasting, as you are skipping meals that were helping to supply you with these vital nutrients and it's important that you replace them. The biggest problem with vitamins and fasting is that taking a vitamin pill in a fasted state may result in stomach pain, nausea and diarrhea. To avoid these unpleasant, unsettling effects, try and get your vitamins down while in the fed state. If this is impossible, try taking your vitamins at night so you can sleep through the discomfort.

Alternatively, you might choose vitamins in liquid form, as they are easier to digest while fasting. If you don't normally take vitamins, a basic multivitamin that provides 100% of your daily intake is a great start to ensure you aren't missing out on anything while intermittently fasting.

Why would anyone fast who doesn't want to lose weight?

It may seem odd to someone who is considering intermittently fasting in order to lose weight, for anyone who has their weight under control to change their eating habits or patterns. After all, aren't they already living the dream? Let's not forget about all the other benefits of intermittent fasting:

- Fasting for athletes: Fasting offers a consistent method of fueling and resting the body that works under many of the same principles as training and rest days. It offers them a much more convenient way to ensure that they consume the food they need to train than the other option of eating small meals every 2 or 3 hours, and it allows them to maintain a nutrition routine that provides a lengthier feeding time which can be enjoyed with friends and family.

- Fasting for health benefits: There are people who swear by fasting because they feel it improves their sleep, mental clarity, and helps them control and maintain chronic diseases such as diabetes, cardiovascular disease, multiple sclerosis, fibromyalgia, chronic fatigue syndrome, cancer and the side effects from chemotherapy.

- Fasting for busy people with poor eating habits: People who travel a lot for business often end up feeling less than well most of the time, due to poor eating habits developed as a result of airport restaurants and late-night vending machines. Establishing a consistent intermittent fasting schedule, including preplanned but convenient and portable food items, allows for much better nutrition, and often fits in well with lengthy travelling times.

- Fasting for financial health and wellness: Which of these two scenarios sounds like a better way to save money? Buying cheap prepared foods like ramen noodles, frozen pizzas and hamburger helper and eating them 24/7 at will, or fasting for 16 hours a day, then eating fresh homemade salads, cooked beans, whole grains and chicken during your eight-hour feeding window? I rest my case.

How should I prepare myself to fast intermittently?

Before embarking upon an intermittent fasting program, it will help to mentally and physically prepare for the challenge ahead. There's definitely a mindset process involved in successful intermittent fasting as well as some practical physical considerations.

- Consult your medical practitioner before beginning ANY new eating program. This is standard boilerplate language, but there's a reason for it – it's a necessary step if you are going to embark on intermittent fasting in an informed, safe manner.

- Make sure you are well-hydrated and avoid salty or sugary foods before you fast.

- Don't stuff yourself the night before you fast. This "last supper" mentality is a rookie mistake that will give you indigestion, a poor night's sleep and an even ruder awakening to your stomach and brain when you follow up the preceding evening's bacchanalia with a fasting period.

- Mentally prepare: Remind yourself several times that you are not going to starve to death – that intermittent fasting is a measurable period of time that you have CHOSEN not to eat within. The first step is fasting. The second is feeding. The third step? Repeat!

- Develop an intermittent fasting mindset: Here's the thing – if you start a fasting period and 5 minutes into it you're thinking, "I'm never going to get through this – I'm already hungry and I can't do this." Guess what? You know the answer. If, however you start a fasting period and 5 minutes into it you're thinking, "I'm feeling strong. I don't eat when I sleep for hours and hours. I know I can do this", chances are, you will in fact succeed. In the words of sociologist William Thomas, "If men define situations as real, they are real in their consequences." Interestingly, this holds equally true for both of the mental scenarios above!

What should I eat to break my intermittent fast?

The basic philosophy behind beginning a feeding after an intermittent fasting period is to eat as if you had never fasted to begin with, or forget about the fasting period and carry on normally. That said, it's always interesting to try and define "normal". Remembering your intentions for intermittently fasting in the first place can be a great help when planning the meal you will break the fast with.

If your intention is to lose weight by fasting intermittently, then you should break your fast with a moderate meal full of nutrient dense, healthy food that fuels your intention without out flooding it with tons of empty calories. If your intention is to support your athletic training regime by fasting intermittently, then you should break your fast, especially after a fasted training, with 30 to 50% of your allotted daily calories, to replenish and fuel your physical activity.

If your intention is to improve your overall health and wellness by intermittently fasting, you should break your fast with clean, organic whole foods that support your intention and have specific nutritional benefits that jive with your specific health challenges. If your intention is to save time and/or money by intermittently fasting, then you should break your fast with a frugal but healthy food selection that has been prepared in a manner that allows you to eat with a minimum of monetary expenditure and/or further fanfare.

Why do I get headaches when I fast and how can I stop them?

Complaints of headaches especially when beginning an intermittent fasting program are quite common. If you are waking with a headache, you may not have hydrated yourself enough the night before. Sleeping with a carafe of water and a glass beside your bed can help remedy this situation. Not drinking enough water is generally one of the biggest culprits of headaches during fasting and water should be imbibed throughout the fasting/feeding process. And remember: we get about 40% of our daily water needs from the food we eat, so it makes perfect sense that you need to replace that water during intermittent fasting periods. Headaches can also be a side effect of the detoxing process that occurs in intermittent fasting and will be especially prevalent in the beginning stages of incorporating the program into your health regime.

Caffeine in the form of black coffee or green tea can be your friend in this case as long as you drink it in moderation and are not hypersensitive to the jittery side effects of caffeinating. A headache during intermittent fasting could also signal a need for more salt, which can be remedied by drinking bouillon or adding more salt to your food during feeding periods. Finally, a headache during intermittent fasting could be signaling low blood sugar, and if they continue despite trying all the tricks and tips above, you should consult your doctor and have your blood sugar tested.

Isn't intermittent fasting just a fancy way of saying I'm starving myself?

In a word, NO! You are voluntarily choosing to refrain from eating for a finite period of time of not more than a total of 48 hours in a seven-day period. Let me bring the actual scientific facts of the process of starvation in to help me convince those of you who still don't believe me...

The Process of Starvation

- **PHASE ONE: After three days,** fatty acids are used by the body as an energy source for muscles, but lower the amount of glucose that travels to the brain. Fatty acids also include a chemical called glycerol that can be used, like glucose as an energy source, but it too, will eventually run out.

- **PHASE TWO can last for up to weeks** at a time. The body mainly uses stored fat for energy. A breakdown occurs in the liver and turns fat into ketones, which are groups of three water-soluble molecules. The brain uses these ketones for energy along with any remaining glucose. At this point the body slows down the breakdown of protein.

- **PHASE THREE:** Fat stores are depleted and the body turns to stored protein for energy, breaking down muscle tissue. The muscle tissue breaks down very quickly. When all sources of protein are gone, cells can no longer function.

- **DEATH BY STARVATION** is usually from cardiac arrest, an infection or other result of tissue breakdown. The body does not have the energy to fight off bacteria and viruses. Generally, it takes **8 to 12 weeks** to starve to death, although there have been cases of people surviving **25 weeks or more**.

Now then... my apologies if this seems a bit brutal, but I think I've graphically shown the difference between intermittent fasting and starvation.

I've heard intermittent fasting isn't safe for women... What are the facts?

Women are more hormonally sensitive than men. Because of this, they may respond more intensely to the challenges of intermittent fasting, and need to consult with a medical professional before starting an intermittent fasting program, especially if they have menstrual and/or fertility issues. Once intermittent fasting has been undertaken, women should also pay special attention to their menstrual cycle, and seek medical guidance if they begin missing periods.

There is a modified or "crescendo" technique of intermittent fasting that will help women who experience hormonal sensitivity. This is a more gradual approach that will help the female body adapt to fasting. Here are the basic rules:

- Fast on 2-3 nonconsecutive days per week
- On fasting days, stick to light workouts such as yoga or light cardio
- Fast for 12-16 hours
- Save strength training for feeding periods or feeding days
- Drink loads of water
- After a few weeks, add another day of fasting and monitor how it goes.

Why can't I have a protein shake when I'm fasting?

Because protein shakes are a MEAL replacement option! Even though they are marketed for their nutrient-density, are packed with protein, are convenient and easily digestible they are, technically FOOD. You can't eat food when you are intermittently fasting – hence you can't drink a protein shake. People get confused about protein shakes – check out diet, fitness, and nutrition and health websites if you don't believe me. I used to shake my head in wonder when I first saw this question asked.

Now I've had a change of heart and have decided to educate rather than ridicule! If you look at the nutrition label on a protein shake you will see that they contain anywhere from 100 to 300 plus calories a shake. If you are on a 5:2 type of intermittent fasting program and you are consuming 500 to 600 calories on your "low" days, feel free to indulge in one or 2 of these shakes if they don't bring you over your total calorie count. If you are on Whole Day Fasting or in the fasting portion of your Time Restricted intermittent fasting cycle don't even think about it!

How can I fast when I'm on vacation?

I indirectly referred to the answer to this question when I was explaining some of the advantages of Whole Day Fasting and 5:2 Intermittent Fasting. Because you are confining your fasting to 2 non-consecutive days of the week, you can automatically end up with a 4-day feeding unit of time. This will help the eating challenges of holidays and vacations in a big way. Another option would be to switch to time restricted intermittent fasting during vacations and holidays, so that there is an 8-hour period during each day for you to eat socially and/or indulge a bit. It might be fun, also to think outside of the traditional food-centric box for a moment, and plan a holiday or vacation that isn't all about overindulging.

Sign everyone up for a half marathon or a day's biking or hiking tour! It's easier to stick to intermittent fasting during festive times if you have company doing it. Finally, giving yourself a week or two break from intermittent fasting doesn't need to be the end of the world. As long as you get back to plan sooner than later, you'll be back in business before you know it and no worse for the break.

Can intermittent fasting really be a long-term weight loss solution?

Honestly, I believe that intermittent fasting is THE solution for long-term weight loss! My reasoning is that because it is NOT a diet, but a lifestyle choice with flexible options, intermittent fasting can be a vital part of the rest of your LIFE. I've already established that this is a sustainable, flexible, balanced, cost-effective timesaving way to incorporate healthy weight loss into your health regime. I've also touted the additional health benefits, including better sleep, mental clarity, increased longevity and preventative protection against a host of chronic diseases caused by poor diet and overindulgence. There is no time limit on intermittent fasting; it will flex and accommodate your health and nutrition needs throughout your weight loss journey and onward through future weight maintenance challenges.

Can I stop fasting once I reach goal weight?

Of course, you can...but WHY would you? If you have taken the time and effort to acclimate yourself to intermittent fasting AND it helped you achieve your personal weight loss goal, why would you go BACK to "diet-think" and stop the program once you reached goal? This type of thinking and finite goal-driven weight loss systems that were devised around this philosophy is precisely WHY people generally don't tend to keep the weight off and worse still, WHY they not only gain back the weight they originally took off, but bounced at the bottom like a trick yoyo and catapulted up to new weight highs!

Think of intermittent fasting programs like this: The constants, or boundaries of these plans are the FED state and the FASTED state of being. These are both natural states for all human beings, and as a matter of fact, human beings are constantly in either one state or another. So why not regulate these states? This is where the variables, or flexibility options come in. By regulating how long you are in the fasted state vs how long you are in the fed state, you can control how long your body ingests and digests food and how long your body rests, burns stored energy sources and detoxes and repairs. You regulate these times, and you can adjust them to your personal needs and goals.

Following an intermittent fasting program that automatically provides you with a consistent, sustainable set of nutritional boundaries, within which you can vary how much and what kinds of food you want to introduce to your body, depending upon and balancing between your needs and desires. In the end, as with so many sustainable platforms, it comes down to balance. Finding and establishing balance are the hard parts of the equation. With the help of intermittent fasting, maintaining this balance becomes manageable and sustainable throughout a lifetime.

Common Fasting Mistakes And How To Avoid Them

At this point I am more than a bit hopeful that you, too are ready to begin your intermittent fasting journey. But, before you start, I've listed some of the mistakes people make while fasting as well as ways you can avoid making them too.

Quitting before you give intermittent fasting a fighting chance:

It's a lifestyle! Yes - it's a challenging transition but the potential rewards are AMAZING! I've read many an account of people who have basically fasted for two and half hours and called it quits. For Pete's sake, everyone can fast for at least 6 hours right out of the box. How do I know that? Because even the worst sleeper (have I mentioned that intermittent fasting can improve your sleep?) has had a "restful" 6 hours of sleep every once in a while. One of the most visceral accounts of this "quitting out of the gate" mentality was a man who journaled about preparing for his first intermittent fast. I read with growing interest, as he parroted back his positive research findings, added up all the potential benefits, and ate his last meal in preparation for the BIG event. He literally wrote about the first couple of hours then stopped.... In the middle of a sentence! It was like, "I'm now twenty minutes into my second hour and I have to say ..." That's all he wrote! I laughed out loud, but

I also felt kind of sad for him. Sad for the missed opportunity. Sad that no one told him to take intermittent fasting at his own pace. Sad that he felt like he had failed again and probably "rewarded" himself by eating everything in the kitchen cupboard.

I'm going to ask you to please give intermittent fasting at least 30 days – one month to try it out and experience the changes it makes. And please don't limit yourself only to pounds lost. Take measurements every week. Journal how your sleep is and how your energy ebbs and flows. Write about your food choices and how you feel about the food you eat after a fasting period. Are you drawn to new and/or different foods than you have been in the past? Has the amount you eat changed? How often are you eating during feeding periods? At the end of the 30 days, put it all together. I think you'll be pleasantly surprised that you did, and I'll be shocked if you're not!

Going whole Hog on your first fast:

There is no humiliation in easing into intermittent fasting. Take advantage of the many different intermittent fasting plans in existence and "date" a couple of them before making a big commitment. You may find that several plans resonate more than others, and want to mix and match plans or create your own hybrid. Just remember the golden rules: No more than two 24-hour period fasts per week, and no two 24-hour fasts on consecutive days. For time restrictive plans, don't go more than 16 hours each day without feeding for the balance of the 24 hours.

Alternatively, design your own gradual immersion schedule to acclimate yourself to intermittent fasting gracefully. You could accomplish this either by gradually extending the periods you fast or by gradually decreasing the hours you feed. The choice is yours as long as the goal of intermittent fasting remains authentic and the golden rules are adhered to.

Eating as much crappy food as you can!

So, you've been intermittently fasting religiously. You've got the timing down to the second and you never cheat...during the fast. But when it's feeding time...Souie!!! All bets are off and any indulgence is fair game. Okay. Deep breath. Let's have a reality check. Are you really surprised you haven't lost much weight, or you don't feel so great or you're experiencing a lot of gastric distress? It is an amazing fact about human beings: we can take pretty much any "best practice" and warp it right out of recognition! It doesn't matter how good you are at the fasting part if you put bad gas in your tank at the end of the day. Here's a good rule of thumb if you're having a hard time coming to terms with the fact you can't eat like a drunken frat boy and lose weight by fasting intermittently:

Just because you CAN (eat like a lumberjack) doesn't mean you SHOULD.

You sit around and wait for the results...
Basically, especially when you first start intermittently fasting, it's highly advisable to keep your mind and body doing something so you don't sit around obsessing on the fact that you can't eat. Don't clear your schedule for your first fast. Live your life and let it fill you instead of food. Try and schedule activities that aren't about food in any way. Don't tempt yourself by hanging around people who can (and will) eat. Avoid break rooms and snack cabinets at the office. Take a miss on the third birthday party cake-fest this week! Give yourself a break and take a nice long walk. Watch your favorite comfort show on Netflix or give yourself permission to take a well-deserved afternoon nap. You will be amazed, and perhaps a bit startled by how much food there is in western culture; how we idolize it, covet it and include it every time we gather to mark an important event; be it a joyous wedding or a somber funeral. It will give you pause – take that pause to reflect and decide how much you want food in your life.

Going overboard with the "stimulants":
So, caffeine in the form of coffee and tea is totally allowed when you intermittently fast and that's a good thing. But, you know what they say about too

much of a good thing... Remember the whole balance thing so your pleasant morning coffee "euphoria" doesn't turn into a raging case of café nervosa! Too much caffeine will wreak havoc with your stomach and your nervous system. Drink coffee and tea mindfully, always keeping your personal tolerance levels in mind.

Fearing "the hunger":
Learn to recognize and come to terms with casual hunger. Know, with the growing assurance that comes with acclimating yourself to intermittent fasting, that casual hunger is a passing thing. You have the knowledge to understand that short term fasting doesn't cause the body to "devour its own" muscle tissue or cause any other bodily harm. Don't let your mind play games with your intentions.

Overtraining:
While it's true that you might get away with intense workouts on fasting days, why take the chance of overextending or even injuring yourself? It is a simple fact that you will most likely feel better if you give your body a bit of a break on fasting days. Experts recommend taking a miss on long aerobic or cardio workouts on days when you are taking in less fuel. Try a more replenishing session of yoga or stretching instead, to prevent

the discomfort and worry of dizziness or weakness.

Ignoring body temperature changes when fasting:

Some people experience an internal temperature drop when fasting. This is a stress response so respond to it. Dress warmly and don't push yourself in any way that would add additional stressors to your day.

In terms of intermittent fasting MORE does not equal BETTER:

There is a very good, scientific reason why you shouldn't fast more than two full days a week? Simply put, most benefits of intermittent fasting decline at the full day mark. If you find yourself stretching out your fasting periods past the recommended times, you need to rethink things. This would be a good place to consider the difference between fasting and starvation.

In terms of intermittent feeding LESS does not equal MORE:

Be very careful not to start cutting down on your food intake to see if you can lose more weight faster. Intermittent fasting is about moderation and balance between fasting and feeding. Don't tip this beautiful balance by cheating yourself out of the food you need to stay healthy. If you feel like this might be happening, seek medical help immediately!

Don't stalk the clock:
How ironic is it that the very same people who celebrate the freedom and flexibility that intermittent fasting affords them often fall victim to endless and obsessive clock watching during fasting AND feeding periods. If you fall into this category, try and reinforce the flexibility of fasting by deregulating the exact times you eat during your feeding window. Experiment with snacking. Vary your mealtimes and make allowances for social interaction and special events. Be mindful about developing rigidity around eating. And on the fasting side, if you start or end your fasting period a bit from time to time don't let it ruin your day. Remember, with intermittent fasting every day offers the gift of another opportunity to get your health and wellness right!

Forgetting that it's a cohesive system:
Try not to get caught up in the details of either fasting or feeding. Like the "mind-body connection" that alternative health gurus and personal coaches espouse more and more these days, you can't experience the sum total benefits of intermittent fasting if you don't let the two parts of the plan work together in harmony.

Ignoring what your body is trying to tell you:

At the end of the day, intermittent fasting is only going to be good for you if your body accepts it. If you experience any symptoms besides the slight physical discomforts already discussed, you need to stop the fast immediately. This includes, vomiting, fainting, shortness of breath, panic attacks or any unexpected and/or sudden sharp pain. If you don't experience relief soon after stopping the fast, seek immediate medical assistance.

Expecting Miracles:

Don't get me wrong. I think intermittent fasting is the bomb. Why would I be spending all this time and energy writing this book if I wasn't a true believer? BUT: It is not alchemy or wizardry or magic. Done properly and mindfully, intermittent fasting will help you lose or maintain weight, improve many facets of your general health, save you time and money and provide you with a consistent yet flexible nutrition, health and wellness regime. Here's what it won't change:

The negative effect of eating too many of the wrong calories
   o **How big your muscles get if you don't exercise enough or in the correct way**
   o **Junk food into healthy food**

o **Burning the candle at both ends, by working all day and partying all night**
o **The fact that you are in the end, "only human", and vulnerable to the ups and downs of this crazy thing we call life!**

A Selection Of Intermittent Fasting "Hacks"

In the interest of giving you the best insight and advice to begin your intermittent fasting journey, I have endeavored to search high and low for helpful tricks and tips to make your experience as productive, user-friendly and successful as possible. Herewith are my findings!

- Start small: There's no such thing as doing too little when it comes to introducing yourself to intermittent fasting. Something as small as shifting your mealtimes by an hour at a time is a step in the right direction
- Keep it simple: Sometimes you fast. Sometimes you feed.
- Focus on flexibility: Rather than getting upset about not eating, focus on the flexibility of intermittent fasting and how much time you are allowed to eat in moderation rather than being on a relentlessly restrictive diet.
- Remember who you are: Be mindful of your likes and dislikes, hopes and fears, personal lines in the sand. In the end, you need to drive the intermittent fasting bus –not the other way around!
- Be prepared for fasting ups and downs. Remember that this is a lifestyle change as well as a change in ingrained habits. Not

easy but not beyond the realm of possibility.

- Remember your goals, but appreciate the process. This is going to take time, so you need to appreciate the journey and not keep asking, "Are we there YET?"

- Learn to listen to your body. Figure out the difference between physical hunger and mental hunger that just might be looking for things beside the instant gratification of food.

- Appreciate the breaks in your routine. Notice how it feels not to have to have to prep a meal or feel obligated to eat at a culturally prescribed time of day.

- Educate yourself about healthy food. Read up on nutrition or go to your local farmer's market and listen to what the experts have to say about their wares.

- Reflect on how much you exercise and why you do it. Listen to your body if it's telling you to stop or urging you to continue an activity.

- Try to be more productive in the morning. Take advantage of when you are fresh from a good night's sleep to accomplish challenging or complicated tasks.

- Don't tell people you are fasting. People can be negative or skeptical about alternative health practices, no matter how ancient or practical these practices are.

- Indulge sometimes! You are working hard for the greater good of your body. Splurge on dessert every once in a while, to keep yourself in balance. When you eat to live you still have to remember what life is all about!

- Leave your house: If you are living with other people, chances are there are gastronomic temptations behind every door and in every drawer. Give yourself a break and head out for a diverting adventure when you are fasting.

- Make sure your next fast-breaking meal is close at hand. There is no excuse for having to make poor food choices because you don't have healthy food available at the end of a fasting period. It's not like it's a surprise after all!

- Intermittent fasting should simplify your day; not complicate it. If this isn't true, something isn't right. Fix it.

- Fasting begins when you finish your last meal of the feeding period. This detail may seem picky, but it matters.

- Develop a "fasting mindset": project in your mind how the day will go, and prepare yourself for distractions and temptations.

- If it works for you, think about people who have survived shipwrecks, plane crashes, avalanches and other disasters and how they managed to live without food for days and weeks. Your fasting period fears should pale in comparison!

- The key to intermittent fasting is mostly mental. If you can stop listening to other people AND the negative voices in your head full of preconceived notions, old wives' tales and urban myths, you will gain the calm clarity necessary to navigate your fasting journey to healthy feeding!

- The better you are at intermittent fasting the less people will care! It's a fact of life that once the novelty has worn off and there's less chance of failure, other people lose interest in the new and different. Always remember it's about and for you. Not anyone else...

- Make sure your fasting plan fits your lifestyle. Earlier in this book I suggested that certain intermittent fasting plans might be advantageous to people with poor diets who travel a lot. The point is, there are enough IF program options out there to make sure the one you participate in works for your life.

- Eat as healthy a diet as you can afford. Budget the money you save by fasting to buy the quality food your body deserves when you are feeding.

- Don't use fasting to get out of things. Just like a new baby or a puppy, you will be tempted to use your new fasting routine to get out of social obligations that aren't at the top of your list. Be honest instead of making excuses. Don't cheapen the good things in your life by using them to avoid unpleasantness.

- Be a life-learner: Keep learning all you can about the science behind intermittent fasting. It's miraculous stuff!

- Don't overeat. If there is one thing intermittent fasting should teach you, it's that there will always be another opportunity to eat. Learning delayed gratification eventually teaches us how to quell the needy voices in our hearts.

- Pamper yourself when you are fasting. Pretend you are at an expensive spa and indulge in a long bubble bath. Get a pedicure or massage. Celebrate your healthy body!

- Time your hunger attacks. Generally, hunger pangs will last around 15 minutes. Drink a large glass of water and check the clock.

- Try the "no liquid calories" challenge. Even during feeding times, see how it feels to cut out all liquid that contains calories, including soda, alcohol, juice, and added cream and sugar to your feeding window coffee and tea.

- When you eat, practice eating slowly. This goes hand in hand with overeating. Delayed gratification is a beautiful thing and no one is going to steal your food if you don't gobble it right down.

- Eat nutrient dense foods first. Protein, fruit, vegetables and nuts should get top priority. Save the fats and sugary treats for last. You will end up eating less of them this way.

- Eat when you are hungry during feeding windows. Retrain yourself to really listen for physical hunger and relearn how to take cues from your body and eat with mindfulness and authenticity.

- Change your feeding window. Is there a big food-themed party looming in your future? Fear not! Change that day's feeding window time, and *bon appetit*!

- Save your indulgences for eating with others. When you eat alone, be strict with your intake. This will allow for more flexibility and treats when eating with others.

- Track your results. Tracking is useful in helping you figure out what's working and what's not on your intermittent fasting adventures, and will help you decide where to make adjustments and modifications.

- Once you have gained confidence, embrace your difference and share your intermittent fasting experience with others. This is still nutritional pioneer territory for a lot of people and as long as you are sure of yourself, you need to share the wealth!

- Stay positive for the long haul. Some say that we are creatures of habit. I would like to amend that statement. I believe we are creatures of bad habit. Making positive changes and sticking to them doesn't always seem to work for humans in the long run. Be on the lookout for old nutritional habits that start poking their tired old noses into new lifestyle choices, when we least expect it or when we are dealing with stress. Understand that just like a person who hasn't smoked in 20 years can light up after hearing bad news, a person who has been faithfully following a solid intermittent fasting regime can very easily pick up a fork, seemingly out of the blue and stick it right into a forgotten junk food indulgence just as fast. When and if this happens, it is more important to recognize the action, figure out what made it happen and then move on, instead of feeling like a failure and eating like one too.

- Here's a great rule to intermittently fast by: You can occasionally eat a "cheat" meal, but you can NEVER cheat by eating during a fasting period!

Establishing New And Healthy Eating Habits

If you google how long it takes to establish a new eating habit, you generally get 21 days as the answer. Where did that number come from? My research says it was determined in the 1950s by a plastic surgeon named Maxwell Maltz who noticed that his patients became accustomed to their new looks in about 21 days. So, there you go! Anyway, in the spirit of intermittent fasting being a lifestyle choice AND a lifelong choice, I say let's not put an arbitrary number on change. Let's make it part of the journey; part of the process.

I think one of the best benefits intermittent fasting offers is the opportunity to establish new and healthy eating habits for the following reasons:

- Intermittent fasting allows you to viscerally experience how the mindful consumption of food affects the fasted body. Each and every day becomes a chance to tweak how and what you fuel your body with, as well as to experience, in real time, how your body reacts to that choice.

- Intermittent fasting gives you the boundaries and support system to learn how to balance food consumption with how efficiently your body utilizes the energy it receives from eating.

- Intermittent doesn't put a time limit on your health, only on your fasting and fed states!
- Intermittent fasting literally GIVES you time, in the form of the fasting state, to reflect on your food choices and make better plans and choices.
- Intermittent fasting has no dependence upon expensive, hard-to-find, and/or exclusive products or ingredients to guarantee its efficacy. You do not need to have any sort of wealth to practice intermittent fasting. In truth, it can be a healthy option for frugal living.
- Intermittent fasting offers a complete system of food management, that can flex to the changes you will experience throughout your life.

Now let's focus on the fuel that energizes intermittent fasting; the food that gives this process viability as well as vitality. Here are some healthy food choices, grouped by the recommended order in which they should be consumed when breaking a fasting period.

- Healthy Protein Options: Seafood; white-meat poultry; milk, cheese and yoghurt; eggs; beans; pork tenderloin; soy; lean beef; meal replacement drinks; cereal or energy bars

- Healthy Fruit Options: Mango; pomegranate; guava; raspberries; oranges; apples
- Healthy Veggie Options: Kale; Brussels sprouts; broccoli; bell pepper; artichokes; spinach
- Healthy Fat Options: Avocados; walnuts; nut and seed butters; olives and olive oil; ground flaxseed; dark chocolate
- Healthy Carb Options: Oatmeal; yams; brown rice; whole grains and whole grain breads and pastas; couscous; quinoa; pumpkin; butternut squash

Eating the first fast-breaking meal in this order ensures that nutrient dense food satisfies and fills you first, instead of sugary, salty, fatty processed food that will stuff you with empty calories and cravings!

Using Your Hand To Portion Your Food

I personally find portioning to be one of the ongoing challenges of my life, basically because I enjoy eating large amounts of food at one sitting! No matter how many times I "educate" myself about portion size and control, I am constantly visually stunned by how small many "normal" single sized portions are. But that's my sad... When I am being mindful, I search out single-serving size items of food as often as I can, sacrificing savings and choice for the comfort of having someone else portion my food appropriately. But there is a better way! You can actually use your hand to figure out units of food! Here's how to do it.

Note: This system was devised to give appropriately sized portions for people who want to lose weight. If you do not need to lose weight but still want a system of measuring your food, you can still use this technique and eat more units per meal.

Protein portions = your palm. One unit of protein should be the size of the portion of your hand between your fingers and your wrist.

Fruits and veggies = the size of two fists. One unit of fruits and/or veggies should be the size of your two clenched fists arranged together at the fingers, ending at the wrists.

Good fats = your thumb. One unit of good fat should be the size of your thumb, from its tip to where it meets your palm.

Healthy carbs = your fist. One unit of healthy carbs should equal the size of one of your clenched fists, ending at the wrist.

This method came from Isagenix, and I think it's pretty foolproof for accuracy and the simple fact that it's impossible to lose your measuring tools! If you arrange your plate of food using this method, and you are counting calories, one meal should come in at a total of 400 to 600 calories. This also gives the non-weight-loss folks a good gauge of their food units and lets everyone keep a "hand"le on portion control. Sorry!

Time and/or Money Saving Meal Preps

Saving money and/or time are major benefits that

can be realized when intermittent fasting. Utilizing the following tricks and tips will also simplify and streamline your intermittent fasting process. Win. Win!

- Buy beans and whole grains in bulk. Beans, oatmeal and other dried whole grains such as brown rice, quinoa and couscous can be an inexpensive source of quality health food when purchased in bulk from supermarkets or large health food stores*

- Cook dried beans and whole grains in a modern pressure cooker. Today's safe, efficient stovetop and electric pressure cookers or instant pots make quick work of cooking dried beans and whole grains like steel cut oatmeal. What used to take an overnight soak and hours of cooking time can now be accomplished in under an hour, giving you enough delicious protein and healthy carb sources for a week's worth of meals in one cooking session. You can use more expensive meat, poultry and fish sources as a condiment to your meals, adding flavor while saving money.

- Pre-portion your food units. Using the hand method explained previously, portion out your food for a week or more at a time and refrigerate or freeze as necessary. I find double zipper sandwich bags to be perfect for this prep.

- Buy 1-pound packages of meat (preferably when on sale). Cut the meat into 4 equal portions, stick each in a sandwich bag, seal and freeze. If you buy 1 pound each of pork, steak, chicken and salmon and prep it this way, you end up with 16 meal portions in 5 minutes!

- Buy local meal services. If cost is not a primary concern, and you are new to the intermittent fasting game, have dietary restrictions, need a wakeup call re: portion size and are low on time or inspiration, find local meal service plans, like Paleo or vegan specialists. The price for 5 meals can be pricey, but the convenience, portion size, nutrition info and culinary prowess and imagination you get can be priceless.

- Set a schedule: work a one-day a week food prep session into your intermittent fasting regime.

- Have the right appliance for the job: keep these time and money-making appliances at the ready for quick and easy feeding meal prep: rice cooker; crock pot; pressure cooker; outdoor grill; Foreman indoor grill; microwave oven.

- Get food wraps, bags and containers at the dollar store. Stock up on all your food prep accessories at these handy discount stores.

- Buy a personal cooler or thermal lunch bag. Buying healthy meals at a restaurant, deli or salad bar can be frustrating and expensive. Bring your food to work and social activities and enjoy the savings as well as guilt free eating!
- Prepped meals are more convenient and definitely better for you than fast food. What's faster than fast food? Prepped meals waiting patiently in your fridge. What's better for you than fast food? Just about anything...
- Spice up your life with seasonings and salts: Nothing puts excitement into basic prepped meals like the addition of fresh or dried herbs, spices and seasonings during the prep and cooking processes. Experimenting with the many differently sourced salts available on the market day will also punch up the flavor of food and add sodium, if you are depleted, to your feeding windows.
- Seeds and nuts are nature's croutons! Sprinkle seeds and nuts over salads, soups and veggies for the texture and taste boost you'd normally rely on croutons and breadcrumbs for.
- If variety ISN'T the spice of your life and you like eating the same meals over and over, prepping large batches of your

favorites, portioning them out, eat at your pleasure and repeat, and repeat....

- Prep, portion and store your meals in mason jars. You can even heat them up in the microwave, once you've removed the lid!
- Check out YouTube videos for inspirational intermittent "feasting" meal preps.

Nutrient Dense Food Swaps

Sometimes it's hard to find nutrient dense foods that can substitute for old, less healthy food standbys. Here are a few innovative swaps to help you in your quest for good health:

- Nut "cheese" spreads for traditional cheese spreads and dips. These are great as sandwich spreads, as a dip with veggies, stirred into pasta or whole grain dishes or used as a dressing on salads. They are a great way to get heart healthy fats into your regime and make a great substitute for processed, fatty, salty cheese spreads.
- Frozen zucchini or peas for some of the frozen fruit in smoothies. Boost the fiber in your healthy smoothie AND decrease sugars.
- Puréed avocado for mayonnaise. Use anytime you would use mayo, including as a sandwich spread, as a binder in tuna, chicken or egg salad, in deviled eggs, and as

a creamy base for dips and salad dressings. You'll be adding fiber, potassium, healthy fat and vitamin E right along with a great flavor boost!

- Dark, leafy greens for iceberg lettuce. Use a variety of these zippy greens in salads, smoothies and wraps (as wraps, too!) for a hearty serving of vitamin K, E, A, C and B, as well as minerals and fiber. Compared to these leafy superheroes, watery, pale iceberg is the "junk food" of the lettuce world.

- Coconut milk for dairy milk. Great for vegans as well as anyone who wants a great source for good fats. Use anywhere and for anything you would use dairy milk, including coffee, in whipped cream, ice-cream and in soups.

Specific 5:2 Minimal Calorie Day Food Choices

If you have chosen the 5:2 intermittent fasting plan and are initially stumped by how to spend your 500 to 600 calories on the two minimal calorie days, here are some options, broken down by meals and snacks.

Breakfast ideas (all under 200 calories):

- Packet of plain organic instant steel cut oatmeal made w/water and topped with 1 tablespoon of raisins
- 1 cup nonfat Greek yoghurt topped with ½ cup thawed, quartered frozen cherries
- 1 hardboiled egg, with ½ apple sliced and 2 teaspoons all-natural peanut butter.

Lunch ideas (all under 200 calories):

- Avocado toast made with 1 slice of whole grain toast, 1/6 of an avocado, mashed with lemon, salt and pepper to taste, sprinkled with a few sunflower seeds
- Skinny burrito in a jar made with ¼ cup salsa, ¼ can drained black beans, ¼ cup reduced fat shredded cheddar cheese and dollop of nonfat Greek yoghurt
- 1 banana with 10 almonds

Dinner ideas (all under 200 calories)

- Chicken lettuce cups made with 2 butter lettuce leaves, ¼ cup shredded chicken breast, matchstick cucumber and carrots, balsamic vinegar, salt, pepper, fresh mint leaves and 1 tablespoon chopped dry roasted peanuts
- Zoodle primavera made with ¼ large zucchini, ¼ of an orange bell pepper, ¼ cup cherry tomatoes, 1 ½ large kale leaves, fresh oregano and basil, 8 ounces cooked down strained tomatoes, 1teaspoon olive

oil, with herbs, spices, salt and pepper to taste.

- Omelet made with 3 egg whites, 1-ounce fat free cheese, 1 thin slice of lean ham, chopped and ½ diced onion.

100 calorie snack options: 1 cup of blueberries; ¾ ounce of sharp cheddar cheese; 1 roasted skinless chicken drumstick, 2 medium kiwis; 2 medium figs; 10 natural blue corn tortilla chips; 1 small baked sweet potato, 2/3 of an ounce of dark chocolate, 25 dry-roasted, unsalted pistachios; 1/3 cup canned red kidney beans; 9 Kalamata olives; 2 cups of watermelon; 1 cup fresh raspberries.

Meal replacement shakes and bars can also help on low calorie 5:2 days. Just be sure to read the nutrition labels for clean, natural ingredients and so you don't underestimate the calorie count. Finally, remember that using the hand portion method will result in a plate of food that will come in at between 400 and 600 calories, so if you are vigilant with the ingredients you could design a main meal for this day, using this method. I end this chapter with what I think is a very apt quote from Dr. Michael Eades, an advocate and participant of intermittent fasting:

"Diets are easy in the contemplation, difficult in the execution. Intermittent fasting is just the opposite – it's difficult in the contemplation, but easy in the execution."

Conclusion: Putting It All Together

As I come to the conclusion of this book, I have a confession to make. Even as I write these words, I am actively experiencing a Whole Day Intermittent Fast! Although I have been an advocate and an active participant of and for intermittent fasting as a life choice and lifestyle for quite some time, researching and writing this book has given me a lot of "food for thought". I hope it has done the same for you.

My intention in writing this book was to immerse the reader in all things relating to intermittent fasting – to offer a primer in this ancient, yet currently trending and ever more popular health and wellness regime. I believe that intermittent fasting is so popular (and has been since the turn of the millennium) because it is grounded in common sense and based upon a physiological cycle that already occurs in each and every one of us: the cycle of the fasted vs the fed state. When we embark on the journey of intermittent fasting we are simply regulating the time that passes between when we feed and when we fast. If you think about western civilization and how plentiful and convenient our food sources have become, paired with how little most of us have to physically expend ourselves to procure it, it only makes sense that we are in sore need of an emergency intervention to regulate the resulting overindulgence and underutilization of and to our physical beings. Enter intermittent fasting!

And yet, as I read personal accounts of what a

positive impact this process has had on countless men and women, I am also struck by how "radical", "extreme" and "out there" intermittent fasting is still perceived by many. Even some of its fiercest advocates and active participants caution in their blogs and articles, not to tell people that you intermittently fast, or, if you insist on being the "strange" one in your crowd and sharing your lifestyle choice, to expect ridicule, derision and skepticism in return for your evangelizing and good intentions. It's important to understand that most of this negative reaction is based upon fear and ignorance. People who don't know better are afraid of fasting. People who haven't been exposed to world religion or medical history or alternative health practices are ignorant when it comes to a health and wellness plan that doesn't docilely float along down the "main stream".

If you purchased this book to learn more about intermittent fasting, I congratulate you for your open mind and forward thinking! As you near the end of this book, I have great hope and anticipation that you have gained a greater understanding about what intermittent fasting is, how it works as a nutrition, health and wellness tool and how it can improve so many elements of your life.

I've covered a lot of material in a relatively brief amount of space, so let's review the highlights. If you have read this book in its entirety and reflected upon its information through the lens of self-improvement, the outcomes should include:

- Understanding the religious, cultural and medical history of this ancient practice
- Understanding the science behind intermittent fasting, including the cellular, hormonal, and systemic impact it can have within the human body
- Comprehending the spectrum of benefits intermittent fasting can offer its active participants, including physical, mental, spiritual, quality of life, behavioral, fiscal, time-saving and personal growth improvements.
- Learning about the flexibility of intermittent fasting through reading about three major types of IF: Whole Day Fasting; 5:2 Intermittent Fasting and Timed Restricted Fasting, but understanding that other methods also exist, as well as hybrids and variations, and that there IS an intermittent fasting program that will resonate with you, whether you follow it completely, or further customize it to your specific needs and desires.
- Acquiring the knowledge that Intermittent Fasting can be successfully utilized to target long-term weight loss as well as life-long maintenance after reaching a healthy weight, through continued fasting as well as physical activity.

- That Intermittent Fasting is also advocated for and utilized by individuals who are not primarily looking for weight loss, but who want to reach and maintain other, equally vital health and wellness goals.
- Recognizing that every individual has many questions about intermittent fasting that need to be answered in a comprehensive manner so that the knowledge gained can be implemented and incorporated into their unique process
- Recognizing that there are mistakes that can be made when embarking on the intermittent fasting journey and becoming aware of these potential pitfalls in a preventative manner
- Concluding that intermittent fasting is NOT a diet or has an expiration date – that it is, instead, a way of healthy living that embraces healthy boundaries as well as the flexibility to grow and change with the natural and inevitable ebb and flow of life itself.

As a writer, I have the great honor of also being a teacher and a guide. But perhaps the biggest benefit I get to continuously reap is the ability writing affords me to be an eternal student of life. I truly enjoyed finally learning what metabolism really meant and being able to figure out my TDEE manually, even though it took me an hour to convert the measurements and see where I had messed up my computation! I will sleep a bit sounder tonight knowing if all the information disappears overnight I can still determine how many calories I need to consume a day to maintain my current weight.

When we are young, we get the opportunity to believe in magic a lot, what with fairy tales, and Disney and Christmas and Harry Potter. When we become adults, the magic is harder to locate. My studies into how the body works, the miraculous ways in which it compensates for disease and repairs itself against the damage we and the environment we exist in inflict upon it, has brought magic back into my life. Then, to be introduced to the process of intermittent fasting, a practice that has been followed since ancient times, when the only proof people could amass for its efficacy was through observation and sheer intuition; a practice that has flourished throughout history, coming in and out of fashion, but never completely disappearing only to reemerge at the turn of a new millennium where it could now be judged by cutting edge scientific knowledge and technology – for this practice to not only survive but endure the tests and research and emerge as the ambassador and benefactor of so many health and wellness benefits…. Well. If that isn't MAGICAL stuff, I surely don't know what is!

So thank you. Thank you for joining me on the intermittent fasting journey. I hope I've convinced you to continue the journey and I wish you luck in your future intermittent fasting ventures. I'm also pleased to announce that I've added a BONUS chapter that includes a variable 10-day introductory fasting plan that incorporates lots of the information I've written about in this book. Enjoy!

*BONUS: 10-Day Introductory Fasting Plan!

The following intermittent fasting plan has been designed to include variations on each day for Whole Day Fasting, 5:2 Intermittent Fasting and Timed Restricted Fasting, to accompany whichever of the three plans you have decided to follow. When planning meals for Whole Day Fasting and Timed Restricted Fasting, as well as the feeding days of 5:2, please employ the Hand portion method I described in this book. If your primary goal is to lose weight, please plate each meal you eat, using one of each of the hand portions. If your goal is NOT to lose weight or you feel that you have cut enough calories during your fasting periods, add additional units of "hand" portioned food as you desire, in half or whole units. Also, where physical activity is indicated, go at your own pace, realistically determining your normal level of activity as sedentary, lightly active, moderately active, heavy exerciser or very heavy exerciser. And, of course confer with a medical professional before embarking on the intermittent fasting journey

Day One (Monday):
- **Whole Day Faster:** Good morning! You are only drinking zero calorie beverages today. Don't forget any vitamins and/prescription medicines, if you didn't take them last night. Stay hydrated and if you decide to

work out today, give yourself a break and take it easy!

- **5:2 Faster: G**ood morning! You are only drinking zero calorie beverages today and consuming between 500 and 600 calories. Don't forget any vitamins and/prescription medicines, if you didn't take them last night. Stay hydrated and if you decide to work out today, give yourself a break and take it easy! Try eating five or six 100-calorie snacks, like the ones I listed in the book, interspersed throughout the day and see how that works for you!

- **Timed Restricted Faster**: Good morning! Until you reach hour 16 of your fasting period, you are only drinking zero calorie beverages. Then you will break your fast at hour 16 and eat at will for the next eight-hour fasting period, keeping moderation in mind if weight loss is a goal. If you had an intense workout today, don't forget to consume 30 to 50% of your total daily calories during the first meal you break your fast with. Don't forget any vitamins and/prescription medicines, if you didn't take them last night. Stay hydrated!

Day Two (Tuesday):

- **Whole Day Faster:** Congratulations! You made it through your first whole day fast! How do you feel? Today you are free to eat at will, keeping moderation in mind if weight loss is a goal! Don't forget to "Talk to the Hand" when portioning out your food choices. Feel free to amp up that workout if you wish today. You are in a fed state.

- **5:2 Faster:** Congratulations! You made it through your first 5:2 fasting day! How was it? Today you are free to eat at will, keeping moderation in mind if weight loss is a goal! Don't forget to "Talk to the Hand" when portioning out your food choices. Feel free to amp up that workout if you wish today. You are in a fed state.

- **Timed Restricted Faster**: Congratulations! You made it through your first timed restricted fasting day! How did you do? Until you reach hour 16 of your fasting period, you are only drinking zero calorie beverages. Then you will break your fast at hour 16 and eat at will for the next eight-hour fasting period, keeping moderation in mind if weight loss is a goal. If you have an intense workout today, don't forget to consume 30 to 50% of your total daily calories during the first meal you break your fast with. How's that first meal working for you? If you're having trouble getting all those calories in at one sitting, think about adding a protein shake or eating the meal in shifts! Stay hydrated!

Day Three (Wednesday):

- **Whole Day Faster:** Hey there! It's another day of free eating, keeping moderation in mind if weight loss is a goal! Prep your fasting mindset, for tomorrow is a fasting day. Get a good night's sleep tonight and don't eat too much, too late. Keep feeling the burn exercise wise. You are in a fed state.

- **5:2 Faster:** Hey there! It's another day of free eating, keeping moderation in mind if weight loss is a goal! Prep your fasting mindset for tomorrow is a fasting day. Think about how you want to consume your 500 to 600 calories tomorrow and perhaps, prep for it. Get a good night's sleep tonight and don't eat too much, too late. Keep feeling the burn exercise wise. You are in a fed state.

- **Timed Restricted Faster**: Hello! You're really starting to experience the pattern of timed restricted fasting now. Until you reach hour 16 of your fasting period, you are only drinking zero calorie beverages. Then you will break your fast at hour 16 and eat at will for the next eight-hour fasting period, keeping moderation in mind if weight loss is a goal. If you have an intense workout today, don't forget to consume 30 to 50% of your total daily calories during the first meal you break your fast with. Think about adopting the no liquid calorie rule and only drink zero calorie beverages 24/7. That'll keep you hydrated!

Day Four (Thursday):
- **Whole Day Faster:** Welcome to your second fasting day of the week! You are only drinking zero calorie beverages today. Don't forget any vitamins and/prescription medicines, if you didn't take them last night. Stay hydrated and if you decide to work out today, give yourself a break and take it easy! Why not think about adopting the no liquid calories rule and starting tomorrow, only drink zero calories 24/7? It's up to you!

- **5:2 Faster:** Welcome to your second fasting day of the week! You are only drinking zero calorie beverages today and consuming a total of 500-600 calories. If the snacking worked for you on Monday then go for it. Otherwise try 2 two hundred calorie meals and one snack. Don't forget any vitamins and/prescription medicines, if you didn't take them last night. Stay hydrated and if you decide to work out today, give yourself a break and take it easy! Why not think about adopting the no liquid calories rule and starting tomorrow, only drink zero calories 24/7? It's up to you!

- **Timed Restricted Faster**: Greetings! Until you reach hour 16 of your fasting period, you are only drinking zero calorie beverages. Then you will break your fast at hour 16 and eat at will for the next eight-hour fasting period, keeping moderation in mind if weight loss is a goal. If you have an intense workout today, don't forget to consume 30 to 50% of your total daily calories during the first meal you break your fast with. Today would be a great day to think ahead to weekend plans. Got any brunches or late-night parties looming on the horizon? No sweat. Just shift your 8-hour feeding window to accommodate weekend fun and fast the 16 hours before or after the festivities!

Day Five (Friday):

- **Whole Day Faster:** TGIF and congrats! Look at you with two fasting days under your belt! Today you are free to eat at will, keeping moderation in mind if weight loss is a goal! Plan ahead for weekend fun and try to think where you might go a bit lighter on the food so you can indulge a bit later on. Exercise like you mean it today! You are in a fed state.

- **5:2 Faster:** TGIF and congrats! Look at you with two minimal calorie fasting days under your belt! Today you are free to eat at will, keeping moderation in mind if weight loss is a goal! Plan ahead for weekend fun and try to think where you might go a bit lighter on the food so you can indulge a bit later on. Exercise like you mean it today! You are in a fed state.

- **Timed Restricted Faster**: TGIF and keep on keeping on. Until you reach hour 16 of your fasting period, you are only drinking zero calorie beverages. Then you will break your fast at hour 16 and eat at will for the next eight-hour fasting period, keeping moderation in mind if weight loss is a goal. If you have an intense workout today, don't forget to consume 30 to 50% of your total daily calories during the first meal you break your fast with. Why not try swapping in some mashed avocado for that mayo on your sandwich? So good and so good for you!

Notes and Reflections for ALL Fasters:

Day Six (Saturday):
- **Whole Day Faster:** It's the weekend! Hope you have a fun and active day planned. Today you are free to eat at will, keeping moderation in mind if weight loss is a goal! Pickup football game anyone? You are in a fed state. Why not try swapping in some mashed avocado for that mayo on your sandwich? So good and so good for you!

- **5:2 Faster:** It's the weekend! Hope you have a fun and active day planned. Today you are free to eat at will, keeping moderation in mind if weight loss is a goal! Pickup football game anyone? You are in a fed state. Why not try swapping in some mashed avocado for that mayo on your sandwich? So good and so good for you!

- **Timed Restricted Faster**: It's the weekend. If you've got food-themed plans, go ahead and shift your fasting period and feeding window. Just remember, until you reach hour 16 of your fasting period, you are only drinking zero calorie beverages. Then you will break your fast at hour 16 and eat at will for the next eight-hour fasting period, keeping moderation in mind if weight loss is a goal. If you've made the informed decision to make social, food fun your priority, think about going easier on any workouts. You might need some of those calories at your social gathering!

Day Seven (Sunday):

- **Whole Day Faster:** Sunday already? Don't despair! Today you are free to eat at will, keeping moderation in mind if weight loss is a goal! Go for the Gold, exercise wise. You are in a fed state. Take a moment or two tonight to plan tomorrow's fast. Make sure you've got lots of zero calorie bevs on hand and a to-do list to keep you occupied.

- **5:2 Faster:** Sunday already? Don't despair! Today you are free to eat at will, keeping moderation in mind if weight loss is a goal! Go for the Gold, exercise wise. You are in a fed state. Think about tomorrow's fast and keep tweaking your 500 to 600 calorie menu options if you aren't satisfied or need to mix it up.

- **Timed Restricted Faster**: Sunday already? Did you end up going to that party and watching the sunrise? How's that zero-calorie liquid rule working for you, lol? Ahh well! Today's another day. Until you reach hour 16 of your fasting period, you are only drinking zero calorie beverages. Then you will break your fast at hour 16 and eat at will for the next eight-hour fasting period, keeping moderation in mind if weight loss is a goal. If Today's the day for social, food fun, think about going easier on any workouts. You might need some of those calories at your social gathering!

Day Eight (Monday):
- **Whole Day Faster:** Monday, Monday... You are only drinking zero calorie beverages today. Don't forget any vitamins and/prescription medicines, if you didn't

take them last night. Stay hydrated and if you decide to work out today, give yourself a break and take it easy! Keep busy and enjoy your day

- **5:2 Faster:** Monday, Monday... You are only drinking zero calorie beverages today and eating 500 to 600 calories. How are you spending Today's calorie allowance? If you find yourself on the run, consider a low-calorie protein shake or meal replacement bar! Don't forget any vitamins and/prescription medicines, if you didn't take them last night. Stay hydrated and if you decide to work out today, give yourself a break and take it easy! Keep busy and enjoy your day

- **Timed Restricted Faster**: Monday, Monday... back to the grind. Until you reach hour 16 of your fasting period, you are only drinking zero calorie beverages. Then you will break your fast at hour 16 and eat at will for the next eight-hour fasting period, keeping moderation in mind if weight loss is a goal. If you have an intense workout today, don't forget to consume 30 to 50% of your total daily calories during the first meal you break your fast with. So, what did you think of your first week? Have you lost any weight? Lost any inches? Gained any insight?

Day Nine (Tuesday):
- **Whole Day Faster:** You are rocking these fast days! Today you are free to eat at will, keeping moderation in mind if weight loss is a goal! Workout for all you're worth. You are in a fed state. So, what did you think of your first week? Have you lost any weight? Lost any inches? Gained any insight?

- **5:2 Faster:** You are rocking these fast days! Today you are free to eat at will, keeping moderation in mind if weight loss is a goal! Workout for all you're worth. You are in a fed state. So, what did you think of your first week? Have you lost any weight? Lost any inches? Gained any insight?

- **Timed Restricted Faster**: I don't know about you, but Tuesday's my good news day! Until you reach hour 16 of your fasting period, you are only drinking zero calorie beverages. Then you will break your fast at hour 16 and eat at will for the next eight-hour fasting period, keeping moderation in mind if weight loss is a goal. If you have an intense workout today, don't forget to consume 30 to 50% of your total daily calories during the first meal you break your fast with. What's your favorite protein source? If you've never tried plant-based protein, my advice for you is beans. If you're a beans and greens fan, why not venture into the land of Tofu?

Day Ten (Wednesday):

- **Whole Day Faster:** Time flies when you're on a fast! Today you are free to eat at will, keeping moderation in mind if weight loss is a goal! Keep on truckin'! You are in a fed state. I am so PROUD of you and I hope you are too! Keep referring to this plan if it's worked for you and feel free to continue making it your own.

- **5:2 Faster:** Time flies when you're on a fast! Today you are free to eat at will, keeping moderation in mind if weight loss is a goal! Keep on truckin'! You are in a fed state. I am so PROUD of you and I hope you are too! Keep referring to this plan if it's worked for you and feel free to continue making it your own.

-

- **Timed Restricted Faster**: Time flies when you're on a fast! Until you reach hour 16 of your fasting period, you are only drinking zero calorie beverages. Then you will break your fast at hour 16 and eat at will for the next eight-hour fasting period, keeping moderation in mind if weight loss is a goal. If you have an intense workout today, don't forget to consume 30 to 50% of your total daily calories during the first meal you break your fast with. I am so PROUD of you and I hope you are too! Keep referring to this plan if it's worked for you and feel free to continue making it your own.

All information is intended only to help you cooperate with your doctor, in your efforts toward desirable weight levels and health. Only your doctor can determine what is right for you. In addition to regular check ups and medical supervision, from your doctor, before starting any other weight loss program, you should consult with your personal physician.

FN№

Presented by French Number Publishing
French Number Publishing is an independent
publishing house headquartered in Paris, France
with offices in North America, Europe, and Asia.
FN№ is committed to connect the most promising
writers to readers from all around the world.
Together we aim to explore the most challenging
issues on a large variety of topics that are of
interest to the modern society.

FN№

EASY KETO DIET
KETOGENIC DIET FOR BEGINNERS

BY NATASHA BROWN

All information is intended only to help you cooperate with your doctor, in your efforts toward desirable weight levels and health. Only your doctor can determine what is right for you. In addition to regular check ups and medical supervision, from your doctor, before starting any other weight loss program, you should consult with your personal physician.

The Keto Diet for Weight Loss: Whether You're New to Keto or Not!

Includes delicious meal plans for Keto breakfasts, lunches, dinners and snacks

Introduction

You've probably heard of the Keto diet before, or may even be following it at the moment. It's becoming more and more popular and it's not hard to see why when there are so many success stories out there. Whether you're completely new to the diet or not, this book will equip you with a wealth of extra information that when you put it into practice, will cause the weight to drop off, not only quickly and healthily, but also without feeling tired, lacking in energy, and hungry; feelings you can probably relate to if you've tried other diets.

So why is the Keto diet different from other diets? First of all, there is no calorie restriction. As long as you don't go over your allotted grams of carbohydrates for the day, you can eat whatever you like! You've probably realized by now that it's an extremely low carbohydrate diet and maybe you feel unsure about being able to stick to a diet if you've failed in the past. However, with the keto diet you can be sure to never go hungry. While it can be a challenge to limit your carbohydrates at first; with a few helpful tips, you'll be well on your way to ketosis and fast weight loss. Of course, everyone changing their diet drastically should make sure they run it by their doctor first. You should also be completely committed to taking on the keto diet in order to achieve all the benefits.

This book will prepare you for your journey by explaining the ins and outs of the keto diet and what ketosis is, as well as giving you practical tips to succeed and tips to stay motivated when you hit a plateau or have a social event where you're worried about succumbing to temptation or peer pressure.

There are many reasons why people fail at weight loss attempts. But with a diet like this where if you get peckish you can simply reach for a chunk of cheese or a sausage or two, you'll definitely not feel hungry!

Even after a few days of following the keto diet, many have reported already noticing a difference in their waistline, as well as feeling energized like never before. So, what are you waiting for? You've got an exciting journey ahead of you, and it starts here!

Chapter 1: Keto and Weight Loss

It's important to understand the science behind the ketosis diet as once you know why your body behaves the way it does, you'll feel far more motivated to stick to the right food choices and follow the diet correctly.

Ketosis is the metabolic state your body achieves when your carbohydrate levels are depleted and your body has no choice but to use fat for energy instead. It shows just how amazingly adaptable our bodies are and also raises the question that if our bodies can burn fat for energy, then why do we need to eat carbohydrates at all?

Most of the recommended ratios for how much of each food type we are supposed to eat encourage high amounts of carbohydrates, moderate amounts of proteins and low amounts of fat. We've been programmed for years to think of fats as the devil. The supermarket shelves are lined with products advertised to be low-fat or no-fat, brainwashing us that fats are bad news and to be avoided as much as possible.

The truth is that all these foods you are encouraged to eat lots of and that are low fat; cereals, grains, bread, rice, pasta, potatoes, may not be as good for you as you are led to believe. These foods were introduced to our diets many years ago when humans starting farming and agriculture became more and more a way of life. And then food made its way into factories and we started processing it, adding extra ingredients, and often replacing fat with sugar to make products low fat and 'healthier'.

The question has been raised in recent years, and especially with the growing obesity problems in many countries: Do we have the right idea about what the human diet is meant to entail? The only way to answer this question is to look at the way our bodies process carbohydrates and fats.

So, what happens when you go on a low-fat, high-carbohydrate, calorie-limited diet? Limited fats can leave you feeling hungry, and when you eat again you'll get a boost of energy from the sugar but will soon crash again after it's been depleted in the body. Are you familiar with these energy peaks and troughs? There are so many diets out there because people are still looking for the right way to lose weight. Most diets are hard to stick to, leaving you feeling hungry, tired, and demotivated. It's the reason that so many people give up, sometimes feeling that they are simply meant to be the size they are and that losing weight is simply too much effort.

Now let's think about what happens on a high-fat, low-carbohydrate diet instead. What would you say to a diet that leaves you not only feeling satisfied after every meal, but allows you to eat tasty delicious foods, and also gives you higher concentration levels as well as energy levels? Not only that, but the weight usually drops off a lot faster than with other diets. It might sound too good to be true but numerous people have found just this after following the keto diet.

So, what does the keto diet actually entail? We'll go into more details later but what you need to know for now is that you'll be keeping your carbohydrates down to between 5 to 10 percent of your daily calories, while fat intake will be between 70 to 80 percent and protein between 20 to 25 percent. By following this simple rule and really limiting your carbohydrates you'll easily achieve ketosis and within a few days of following the diet your body will already have started burning fats for fuel and attacking the fat stores in your body. But first let's take a deeper look at ketosis and what actually happens in our bodies.

Chapter 2: What is Ketosis?

As we've already identified, ketosis is when your body uses fat instead of carbohydrates for fuel. This happens when our carbohydrate levels are so low that the body has no choice but to look elsewhere for energy. It starts using the fats that we eat and also the fat stored in our body to burn for fuel instead. This is a process called beta-oxidation and it happens when acetyl-coA levels increase and turn into acetoacetate which then becomes beta-hydroxybutyrate. This may all sound a bit science-heavy but what you really need to know that the by-products of this process are ketones being produced in the liver. They then travel through the bloodstream providing energy to the brain and body.

Scientifically speaking, ketosis occurs when you achieve 0.5mol/L (millimoles per liter) or more in your bloodstream. This can be easily tested by urine strip tests or blood prick tests. This is when you can be sure that your body is in ketosis and is using fat rather than carbohydrates as its energy source. Everyone is different so you might find that you can eat more or less carbohydrates than other people to maintain ketosis and achieve 0.5mol/L or more of ketones in your blood.

It's important to note that high levels of ketones in the bloodstream can be dangerous and that's why you should test your levels regularly, especially if you are new to the keto diet. For this reason, there are some people who believe that maintaining ketosis is unhealthy, but if it's done the right way it can be extremely beneficial.

Ketosis is actually an extremely natural state for the body to be in. Our bodies are designed to burn fat for fuel and naturally operate that way, even when we don't force it that way with our eating habits. Many babies are born in ketosis and it's also used to help those with diabetes and epilepsy. Years and years ago when food was harder to come by than it is now, humans relied on ketosis as a way to get through the winter. During the summer months when food was easier to find, they would fatten up and then these fat stores would be used for energy during the months where food was scarce.

There are two different ways of achieving ketosis but the reason for it is always the same: not enough carbohydrates to burn as fuel. Firstly, we can limit the carbs that we eat through a food plan like on the keto diet. Secondly, if we fast, our bodies will fall into a state of ketosis, and this is often what used to happen to our ancestors during the long winter months.

Nowadays we don't often naturally achieve ketosis, simply because of the readiness of food available; a lot of it being high in carbohydrates. The second you feel a pang of hunger, you don't have to look far in order to be presented with an abundance of choices. The fact that we are so surrounded by food these days makes it difficult to stick to any diet. However, a diet that leaves you feeling hungry makes it even more difficult. Luckily, the state of ketosis actually suppresses appetite, making it easier to resist those high carbohydrate snacks that may have been too tempting to resist in the past.

Chapter 3: How to Start the Keto Diet – What You Need to Know

Now we know that to start burning fat effectively, we need to induce our bodies into a state of ketosis. So, how do we limit our carbohydrates safely?

We've already mentioned the ratio of fat, protein and carbohydrates needed to achieve ketosis but percentages are hard to imagine so let's try to make it a little easier.

The most difficult part of the diet initially will be understanding exactly how much of each food group to consume but the meal plans at the end of the book will help for the first week or so, while you're still getting your head around it all. Those already using the keto diet will find some new recipe ideas to try, which focus on doing keto the healthy way, with plenty of vegetables and fiber, rather than just achieving the correct percentages.

Aiming to eat 70 to 80 percent of our calories from fat might seem like a lot, but remember that fat has more than double the calories per gram compared to protein and carbohydrate. So, let's think about what the target percentages mean in terms of calories for someone who consumes around 2000 per day:

5% carbohydrates = 100 calories or 25 grams
20% protein = 400 calories or 100 grams
75% fat = 1500 calories or 167 grams

It's important to note that dietary fiber is included in most measurements of carbohydrate. Seeing as fiber is a nutrient that we need but that we don't digest, we can take it off our grams of carbohydrates. This will give you a few extra grams of carbohydrates to play with, and also encourages you to eat healthy foods which are high in fiber, giving you more bang for your buck so to speak. The number of grams of fiber can be taken off the total grams of carbohydrate in any food to get to the number of grams of net carbohydrates. This is the figure you are interested in when calculating how many carbohydrates you should be eating.

So, what does 25 grams of net carbohydrates look like? Below are a few approximate examples for different types of food but there is an extensive list later in the book:

Fruit	**Vegetables**
2 apples	7 cups of broccoli
1 banana	5 cups of steamed kale
2 cups of blueberries	2.5 cucumbers
5 dates	1 ½ cups of cooked onion
25 strawberries	8 cups of steamed zucchini

Grains and Cereals

2 ½ slices of bread

2 ½ corn tortillas

2 cups of cornflakes

½ cup of white rice

3/4 cup of cooked spaghetti

Legumes

½ cup of cooked chick peas

1 cup of cooked kidney beans

1 cup of cooked split peas

1 ½ cups of cooked lentils

All the above are approximate measures and it's easy to see that using up your entire carbohydrate allowance on just one food is really easy to do. That's why it's best to avoid foods such as bread, rice and pasta entirely. They take up a huge amount of your carbohydrate allowance for just a small amount. Also, they provide limited nutritional value so it makes a lot more sense to try and use your carbohydrate allowance for lots of vegetables and a limited amount of fruit.

Out of the above foods, vegetables should be where most of your carbohydrate allowance is going to go. You'll need a few more for seasoning, sauces, and the small amounts in some meat and cheese products. However, the intake of most animal products is not restricted. Yes, you read it correctly; on the keto diet, you can eat unlimited amounts of the following:

Chicken	Duck	Salmon
Beef	Quail	Cod
Veal	Venison	Tuna
Lamb	Rabbit	Haddock
Pork	Turkey	Bass

Chicken, meat and fish mostly have no carbohydrates at all if you eat them as they are, completely unprocessed. However, if you're buying deli meats or cured meats you should always check the packaging, as some of them have added sugar or other ingredients and therefore the extra carbohydrates will need to be accounted for. Crabs, lobster, shrimp and other shellfish have a small amount of carbohydrates.

Cheese and dairy products also contain small amounts of carbohydrates but you'll find the higher the fat content, the lower the carbohydrates. Therefore, it's a good idea to switch to cream instead of milk for your coffee and never go for any low-fat options for cheese or yogurt. The best options for dairy products are:

| Eggs | Cheese |
| Thick Cream | Almond Milk |

The other thing to watch out for is condiments. Obviously, things like jams and jellies and tomato ketchup are usually pretty high in sugar. But even when using dried spices and herbs for cooking it's important not to forget to count the grams of net carbs: it all adds up. Some of the lowest carb condiments available are:

Salt and pepper	Ground spices
Vinegar	Hot sauces
Fresh Herbs	Mayonnaise

Almost all oils have zero carbohydrates so that can be a really good way to add fat to your diet and some extra flavor to your food too.

We'll talk more about counting carbohydrates, as well as fats and proteins later in the book, with some lists of foods and some handy Keto swaps, but for now let's keep it simple and look at what a day of eating on the Keto diet might look like, with some basic ketogenic meals.

For breakfast, you might choose to have scrambled eggs made with cream with a couple of spring onions and a tomato chopped up and added to it along with some salt and pepper:

3 eggs
3 tablespoons of full-fat cream
1 tomato
2 spring onions
1 tablespoon of oil
Pinch of salt and pepper

This would have a net carbohydrate rating of about 8.3 grams which is about a third of your daily allowance.

Consider what many would consider a healthy choice for breakfast; maybe a bowl of cornflakes with milk and topped with a few dates:

1 cup of cornflakes
1 cup of milk
1/2 cup of berries

This would have a net carbohydrate rating of about 29 grams! You've already exceeded your allowance on just one meal.

This example shows how important it is to be in the know when it comes to what's in your food. The keto diet is really easy once you get used to it, and are accustomed to shopping and cooking the keto way. However, it takes a little time to get your head around counting carbs, not to mention the fats and proteins too!

For this reason, it's a really good idea to use some kind of calorie counter, especially at the beginning of your journey, but even experienced keto dieters will find it very helpful. You can buy a small book to keep in your bag or desk while you're at work, or otherwise there are many online calorie counters and apps to help you too. Keeping a food diary is also an excellent idea, either in a diary, on a spreadsheet, or using an app on your phone.

So, what could a typical keto lunch look like?

Maybe you choose to have a fried chicken breast with some salad on the side:

1 chicken breast
1 cup of lettuce
1 tomato
¼ cucumber
2 tablespoons of oil
1 tablespoon of apple cider vinegar

This would give you a total of about 8.9 grams of net carbohydrates, which leaves you just 7.8 for the rest of the day. Not sure it will fill you up? Just add another chicken breast, preferably cooked with the skin on to increase the fat content.

However, if you had the same salad but instead of the oil and vinegar dressing chose a honey mustard dressing and added a handful of croutons, you would suddenly be looking at 22.8 grams of net carbs.

A keto dinner could consist of some zucchini noodles fried in oil with pork chops:

2 spiralized zucchinis
Oil
One clove of garlic
2 pork chops

This meal comes to a net carbohydrate rating of about 7.5 grams.

However, if you ate a cup of cooked spaghetti instead of the zucchini you would be looking at a whopping 26.5 grams of net carbohydrates.

It's easy to see how simple changes can have a massive effect on the amount of net carbohydrates you are consuming and this is why it's extremely important to keep a very close eye on your count.

The examples above included lots of vegetables which is important to make the diet as healthy as possible. However, if you are still hungry after consuming your allowed amount of carbohydrates you can simply add extra chicken, meat or other zero or extremely low carbohydrate choices. We'll have a look at lots of different options for meals and snacks later in the book.

Chapter 4: Benefits of the Keto Diet

As you have seen so far, taking on the keto diet takes a bit of thought, planning and preparation. However, when you see the benefits gained from achieving and maintaining ketosis, a bit of extra planning is a small price to pay.

Weight Loss

The foremost benefit and the reason that most people follow the diet in the first place, is the amount of weight that can be lost. And quickly too. Only such low carbohydrate meal plans can boast weight loss in a matter of weeks, which makes it ideal if you have a specific date that you want to lose weight by. And once you've achieved your weight loss goals, you can easily maintain them simply by continuing the diet. Everyone is different and everyone responds slightly differently to how many net carbohydrates they can consume to keep their body in a state of ketosis so you might even find that after you've reached your goal you can up your net carbohydrates slightly. You also might find that you can get away with the odd cheat day, especially if you combine it with intermittent fasting, but more about that later.

So, how does being on the keto diet and getting

your body into ketosis achieve such noticeable and quick weight loss results? The key is increased fat oxidation which is caused when the body burns fat from your diet and also from your fat stores as its primary source. It means that because of not having any carbohydrates available, your body immediately starts attacking your fat cells for energy, which in turn initiates fast weight loss.

Appetite Suppression

When your body is in ketosis you'll notice that you won't feel as hungry as you used to. Many people have reported that they no longer get the mid-afternoon or late-night hunger pangs that they used to. This is due to the fact that burning fat is more consistent than using carbohydrate for fuel. Therefore, you won't experience carbohydrate crashes than cause you to crave sugary snacks. The great side effect of this of course is that it will stop you from overeating and consuming more calories than you need during the day. This can have a huge impact on weight loss.

Increased physical performance

Because your blood sugar levels are more regulated when you're in ketosis, you'll find that your energy levels will stay consistent too, which is great for endurance training and will help avoid crashing. Adapting the body to burn more fat helps the body preserve what glycogen there is in the muscles, which means that the muscle in your body won't be affected, even when losing weight. Also, the fact that oxygen is used more efficiently during ketosis is another reason you may find you're able to train for longer, which is a great side effect!

Increased mental ability

It might surprise you to know that the brain is actually made up of over 60 percent fat. So, it makes sense that eating a high fat diet is going to be beneficial for the brain and its ability. The brain needs a small about of carbohydrates to function but it actually prefers fat for fuel. Ketones deliver energy straight to the brain and because, as we've already said, ketosis enables a more consistent release of energy, you can find that your concentration levels increase and you avoid those slumps of tiredness where you're likely to feel like you need a coffee or an energy boost though eating something.

Other Benefits

It's amazing to see how many benefits the keto diet has, aside from losing weight. Feeling lighter, better able to train and more focused on mental tasks are all great motivators to stick with the diet and are reminders that relying on sugary snacks or coffee to get us through the day are in fact detrimental and not helpful for our energy levels.

There are also a number of medical uses for the keto diet. Children and also some adults with epilepsy are told by their doctors to maintain a ketogenic state in order to control seizures. It has also been known to help with the symptoms of degenerative diseases, such as Alzheimer's and Parkinson's. Cancer patients are often told to cut sugar out of their diets because sugar and carbohydrates feed the cancer, so cutting them out can reduce the growing rate of the tumor. The keto diet as also been used to treat people with diabetes, seeing as it regulates insulin levels in the body.

There has been some bad press lashing out against the keto diet in the past, however, knowing that doctors have prescribed this to many people over the years to help with their illnesses, diseases and medical conditions should alleviate any doubt as to whether the diet is safe and/or healthy. If you have any concern about your health you should definitely speak to your doctor before embarking on the diet and inducing your body into ketosis. Carrying out the diet safely and responsibly and being careful not to let the level of ketones in your blood increase too much can ensure that there will be no risk to your health.

Chapter 5: How to Prepare Yourself for the Keto Diet

You're probably feeling pretty motivated right now. You're reading this book to find out more about the diet and kick start your weight loss, or boost it if you've already started your journey. This chapter is mainly for those new to the keto diet but those already following it will benefit from some reminders about how to stay focused and motivated to stick with it, even when having bad days.

If you've tried to lose weight before you might find that you quickly become demotivated and lose the will power to carry on. You may have had these feelings because you were hungry or tired or feeling down. Or it may have been because you weren't fully prepared to take on the diet and therefore in a moment of weakness you eat something you're not supposed to, or eat too much. It's really important to make a commitment to yourself that you are going to follow the diet and make huge and lasting beneficial changes to your life. So how is the best way to prepare for the diet?

Preparing Mentally

It's a good idea to have a long hard think about

why you want to follow the keto diet. Take out a pen and paper and jot down all the reasons you can think of. It might look something like the following, but try and really do some soul searching and write down everything you can think of.

My reasons for going on the keto diet

- I want to feel comfortable being on the beach this summer
- I want to feel more confident in my body
- I want to feel attractive to members of the opposite sex
- I want to feel energized and positive every morning when I wake up
- I want to be able to run around with my kids/grandkids without getting worn out

Whatever your reasons are, write a list and put it somewhere you will see it on a daily basis. On the mirror in your bathroom or the door of the fridge are good places. You should read through it every morning, like a little mantra to yourself. It will focus you for the day ahead and reinforce the importance of your choices. You may also want to add a couple of photos. One where you felt happy with your body, or maybe of someone who inspires you in life. The other photo should be one that you hate: a photo that maybe made you start your weight loss journey in the first place.

It's very easy to get carried away with life and

forget about your long-term goals, or put them off because you feel like you've got too much on. But you can stay focused by thinking about your weight loss goals and looking at the photos every single morning when you wake up. The reminder will put you in good stead for the day.

Tell People!

Of course, you'll want to share your journey with friends and family, and receive their support and well-wishes. There are a number of reasons it's a good idea to do this.

Once you've made your decision about going on the keto diet, don't keep it a secret! Share your news with as many people as possible. Telling other people with reinforce the decision in your head, and it'll also be embarrassing if you don't succeed, so it gives you some extra motivation to stick with it.

Your new eating habits will also potentially affect those around you. Things are going to change and if you have a spouse or even roommates who are used to sharing the cooking, or shopping with, it's a good idea to take some time to explain to them exactly what you can and can't eat. You're probably going to be eating a lot differently to them from now on.

That also means you're taking your eating habits

completely into your own hands. If you're not used to spending much time in the kitchen this might seem a little daunting, but cooking on the keto diet can be really simple and easy, and we'll go into more about that later.

Planning

It cannot be stressed enough how important planning is in order to succeed on the keto diet. Obviously, there are foods you can pick up on the go when push comes to shove, like deli meats and whole cooked chickens. However, to keep an accurate record of your grams of net carbs per day, it's far better to prepare the majority of foods yourself.

That means making a meal plan for the week ahead and creating a shopping list accordingly.

These are the things that will make your life easier when it comes to planning:

A diary – Invest in a new diary which is purely for keto purposes. You can use it for planning the week ahead and even add in the recipes so when you get home from work you can turn the page to today's date and know exactly what to cook for dinner that night. It'll help you keep organized and make sure you're doing everything you can to maintain your state of ketosis. You can also highlight any upcoming occasions or events where it won't be possible for you to cook and make sure you have freezer options ready for those days.

A journal – Keeping a track of how you feel each day is really important. This goes back to the subject of being mentally prepared as is a great way to track your energy levels and weight loss progress. It can be really inspiring to look back over and give you some motivation if you're having a rough day or you hit a plateau in weight loss.

You don't need to spend too much time on your journal but even writing a few sentences a day will help gage your feelings when you look back. You can even incorporate it into your keto diary if you get one with enough space for planning, recipes, and a short journal entry.

A typical day might look like this:

Breakfast – 3 eggs, 3 bacon, 1 cup mushrooms, scrambled with 1T thick cream (5.5g net carbs)

Lunch – Leftovers from last night – Chicken Cacciatore (7g net carbs)

Dinner – Chili Beef – 8oz ground beef, 1T oil, ¼ diced onion, 1 garlic, 1 chili pepper, 1T tomato paste, 2T kidney beans (9.5g net carbs)

Fry onion garlic chili in oil, add beef, when browned add tomato paste and beans.

Snacks – Smoked salmon (0g net carbs), ½ cup popcorn (2.6g net carbs)

Drinks – Black coffee, tea with almond milk x 2 (1g net carbs)

Net carbs total for day: 25.6g

Felt a bit headachy between breakfast and lunch but it passed when I drank a big glass of water. Need to drink more! Snacked on salmon at night, but more out of habit of wanting to eat anything rather than being hungry. Enjoyed the salty popcorn mid-afternoon. Generally, felt good today, woke up feeling good, just need to drink more water. Excited to weigh myself at the end of the week!

It's a good idea to allot a time each week for planning. You can make your plan and then fill out your diary with your main meals for each day. Pick a time when you're usually not busy, for instance during the weekend, or one lunchbreak during the week. It's good to get into a habit of doing this as it will save so much time when grocery shopping, and will help you keep to your allotted amount of net carbs for the day.

Then after each day you can add any additional snacks and drinks, and work out your total net carbs. You can also write a little about how your feeling and also track your weight loss.

Chapter 6: How to Prepare Your Kitchen for the Keto Diet

Before you start your keto journey, you need to make your kitchen a keto-friendly place. It's no good getting home at night and realizing you haven't anything to eat and then reaching for options that will throw you out of ketosis and massively affect your weight loss potential.

Make a decision and a promise to yourself that you are going to do this. That you are serious. And then clear out your kitchen cupboards. Take absolutely everything out and give away anything that you'll be tempted by. That means bread, pasta, rice, potato snacks, sugary treats, starchy veg, etc. If you're not sure, look up the net grams of carbohydrate per serving size and you will soon have the answer.

If you live with others who are not fellow keto dieters than it might be possible to have your own kitchen cupboard, or shelf in the fridge, so you can separate all the non-keto items.

Once the difficult part is over, the fun bit begins! It's time to go shopping. As well as grocery shopping for your meal plan, which we'll get to in a minute, you'll also want to stock up on some basic supplies: pantry staples that you'll use often and some go to items when you're in a pickle.

The following list is a good place to start but as you get used to the keto diet and develop favorite recipes, you'll adapt your own list of staples.

Fruit

As you've gathered by now, fruit doesn't figure much in your future on the keto diet. However, all things in moderation, of course. You'll only want to eat fruit in very small amounts at a time and it can be difficult to buy fruit in such small quantities so a good option is to buy a bag of frozen berries or rhubarb and keep it in the freezer for occasional use.

Vegetables

You're not going to be eating a hell of a lot of vegetables either, so the same goes with regards to buying too much and then having waste. You'll want to have a meal plan that allows you to use the same vegetables for different meals a few days running. It will cut down on both waste and cost. Batch cooking is also a great idea for using up bigger quantities of vegetables. If you have a big enough freezer it's a really good idea to have a few back-up meals waiting for you. Knowing that you can just pull something out of the freezer and heat it up after a long day at work will also help keep you on the straight and narrow.

Usually a zucchini or two, a bag of lettuce or

arugula, an onion, a few garlic bulbs, a carrot, some celery and some kale is a good place to start for a week's worth of groceries, but for fresh produce it's better to buy to the meal plan rather than stock up as otherwise you'll find produce will get wasted.

Herbs

Freeze-dried herbs are a great option for being able to mix up your options without having to buy fresh all the time. Of course, the perfect option is to grow your herbs yourself so you can snip some off whenever you need, but unfortunately a lot of us don't have the time or space for that. A selection of dried herbs is great in the absence of fresh, but watch the carbs on some of them.

Spices

A few different basic spices are essential to have in your cupboard. Knowing exactly what goes into your food is what's great about the keto diet. You have complete control and you can use flavor to add so much different variety, as well as providing many nutrients and benefits to the body. Spices like cinnamon, chili powder, curry powder, celery salt, and cumin will add flavor to your food without adding many carbs.

Oils

There are so many different oils available and they

can add real flavor to your food and help avoid having to add extra carbs with other flavoring or sauces. Olive oil, avocado oil and sesame oil add a different depth to salads and cooking and can add flavor to the simplest of meals. You'll also want to have some ghee or butter or both in your fridge; essential for that decadent buttery taste, and also gloriously carb free. When struggling to reach your daily intake of calories from fat, adding oil or butter to dishes can really help.

Eggs, Dairy, and Non-Dairy Alternatives

When it comes to eggs, I think it goes without saying that they're a real staple on the keto diet. They're ridiculously versatile and are also low in carbohydrates and high in protein and fat Hopefully you're a fan on eggs as they're a major feature in most keto diet plans. The egg yolk on its own models the keto diet perfectly with its 5% carbohydrates, 75% fat and 20% protein proportions. Make sure you always have fresh eggs on hand, and preferably a few hard-boiled eggs in the fridge too for snacking on.

Unsweetened almond milk or thick cream are the best choices as far as tea and coffee accompaniments go. If you're set on having whole milk then just make sure you really watch your quantities. Cream is great for making quick sauces or little desserts too.

Cheese is another staple, just like eggs. When

reading through keto recipes, you'll soon see that cheese features a lot, and there are many reasons for that. Cheese is low in carbohydrates and high in fats, it comes in so many different types, shapes and flavors, and it also tastes amazing! Just be sure to check the packaging before you buy in case extra carbs have been added. Any self-respecting keto dieter should have at least three different types of cheese in their fridge at any one time: you'll soon find out how good it feels to indulge in guiltless midnight snacks.

Drinks

Everyone likes a tipple from now and then and it's still possible while maintaining ketosis, but not necessarily recommended. Pure spirits like vodka and gin don't count towards our net carbohydrate count, so in effect, they are carb free. But not everyone reacts in the same way and it's best to keep alcohol intake down to a minimum. Judgement is weakened with alcohol so you might find your will-power is affected too which can be bad news when it comes to late night snacks, or hungover breakfast choices. At least in the early days of your keto journey, it's best to avoid alcohol altogether.

As far as sodas are concerned, diet sodas have zero carbohydrates, as well as black tea and coffee. As always, it's important to take care of water intake. On the keto diet this is particularly important because when your body is changing its way of converting energy, a side effect can be dehydration. Buy a refillable bottle and take it with you. Drinking a glass of sparkling water with the juice of half a fresh lemon or lime is a great way to start the morning, and with only 1 gram of net carbs.

Canned Produce

Even though fresh is always better, there are loads of canned items that are useful to have on hand. Coconut milk, tuna, anchovies, beans, lentils, chick peas, tomatoes and tomato paste are all canned goods that come in handy on the keto diet. There are a few vegetables which work well from from cans, such as tomatoes and sweetcorn. Even if you don't use the whole amount in one go, the leftovers can be kept in a fridge or frozen. Therefore, it's a good idea to invest in a few small storage containers too.

Cooking Ingredients

Where would we be without salt? It makes just about everything taste better and it happens to be zero carbs too. It's actually been recommended to up salt intake a little, especially when starting the diet. Dehydration can also lead to a drop in sodium levels so a little extra salt won't do any harm. Buy a nice quality sea salt or pink salt for extra minerals, and it's also a good idea to have some chicken, beef and vegetable stock cubes. There's only 1 gram of carbohydrates per cube and you can even use them to make a quick hydrating and warming drink.

Almond flour is surprising low in carbohydrates compared to corn or wheat flour, however it should still be used in small quantities. Baking soda and baking powder are useful to have, as well as cocoa powder, shredded coconut flakes and peanut butter. Dried corn kernels are nice for the occasional cup of popcorn and you'll probably want a zero-carb sweetener as well.

Nuts and Seeds

The odd quarter cup of chopped nuts is a great addition to salads, stir-fries and curries, as well as enjoying on their own. Buy some jars and keep stocked up with a few different types of both nuts and seeds. Almonds, walnuts, flaxseeds, chia seeds and pumpkin seeds are some good low carb varieties to keep on hand.

Sauces

A great sauce can add a tasty twist to just a few simple ingredients. Favorites include mayonnaise and cider vinegar which have zero carbohydrates. Barbecue sauce, pesto and soy sauce are great when used in small amounts, as well as hummus and tahini.

Meat, Poultry, Fish and Meat Replacements

It's always good to have a varied selection of fresh meats and a few frozen options too. The bulk of your diet is going to be these fat and protein rich foods so you need to make sure you always have plenty on hand, both for cooking and for snacking on. As far as meat is concerned, it's really up to what your preferences are. A big batch of chicken breasts, ground beef or pork, sausages and bacon is a good place to start.

Here is the entire grocery list to get you started. You don't have to buy it all at once, especially if trying to stick to a budget, but over time you should aim to have a kitchen and pantry that include the following:

Lemons/limes – for adding flavor to food and making drinking water more exciting
Frozen berries
Zucchinis – great for spiralized noodles
Lettuce
Arugula
Kale
Onion – use a quarter at a time and keep in an airtight box in the fridge
Garlic
Carrots
Celery
Frozen peas
Frozen herbs – chives, parsley, etc.
Ground cinnamon
Chili powder
Curry powder

Celery salt
Cumin
Olive oil
Avocado oil
Coconut oil
Sesame oil
Eggs
Unsweetened almond milk
Thick cream
Butter
Ghee
Monterey or cheddar
Brie or camembert
Cream cheese
Canned coconut milk
Canned tuna
Canned anchovies
Canned beans
Canned lentils
Canned chick peas – great for making homemade hummus
Canned tomatoes
Canned tomato paste
Canned corn
Himalayan salt or sea salt
Stock/broth cubes
Baking soda
Baking powder
Almond flour
Cocoa powder
Coconut flakes
Peanut butter
Corn kernels

Sweetener
Almonds
Walnuts
Flaxseeds
Chia seeds
Pumpkin seeds
Mayonnaise
Cider Vinegar
Barbecue sauce
Pesto – it's also really easy to make your own
Soy sauce
Tahini
Chicken breasts
Ground beef or pork
Sausages
Bacon
Tuna
Smoked Salmon

So, your pantry is stocked and your fridge is brimming. You're almost ready to start, but there are also a few more items which you may want to invest in to make your kitchen really prepared for keto, if you don't already own them. Here are some items you will definitely find useful:

Scales – So that you can weigh every food and know exactly how much you're eating and therefore work out how many carbohydrates.

Cups – A set of cups is also invaluable for working out portions sizes and many recipes use this measurement scheme.

Storage containers – Jars, plastic airtight containers and tins are really useful for storing pantry items as well as half-used up fruit and veg or leftover meals. You can also save old yogurt tubs and food containers and wash and reuse them to save money.

Cookware – At the very least you'll need a frying pan, a heavy saucepan/casserole pot that can go on the stove and in the oven, and a baking tray, preferably all non-stick.

Knives – If you don't already have a few sharp knives, you should invest in some to keep your sanity in the kitchen. Chopping things with blunt blades is the least fun cooking gets.

Chalkboard – A fun way to motivate yourself in the kitchen, as well as to jot down any pantry items that might need restocking so you can add them to your weekly grocery shopping list.

Spiralizer – If you're a fan of noodles and spaghetti then this is a must-have. Spiralized zucchini is unbelievably similar to pasta, but has fraction of the amount of carbohydrates. It makes a great healthy side dish for any meal and is really versatile too.

There are so many additional kitchen items you can buy that will make cooking easier. The products above are great for starting your keto journey but no doubt you'll want to add more as the time goes on and you become more adventurous with new recipes.

Chapter 7: The Carb List

On the keto diet your main focus should be keeping your carbohydrates as low as possible, and this generally includes eating as much as you like when it comes to meat, chicken, fish, cheese and fats, but limiting intake of fruits, vegetables, legumes, and most of all, grains and cereals. Even when it comes to eating different meats you need to be careful and always check the packaging to see if any sneaky sugar or fillers have been added.

When aiming for ketosis, it's best to look at the net carbohydrate ratings of foods. What does this mean? Well, because the body doesn't digest fiber, we can take off any grams of fiber from the total grams of carbohydrate in the food. All the listings below are for net carbohydrates per serving.

Meat, poultry, fish, and other protein sources

These foods are generally great for those on the keto diet to indulge in freely, however care still needs to be taken as extra grams of carbohydrate can easily creep in, especially when it comes to more processed varieties, such as deli meats and burgers. Therefore, it's best to go for pure meat sources. Not only will you avoid extra grams of carbohydrates but you'll also avoid added ingredients that may not be very healthy. It's best to go for organic as much as possible but obviously that depends on budget too.

All beef, steak, chicken, turkey and fish has zero net grams of carbs so only produce with any carbohydrates are listed below, including some types of seafood as well. However, a few zero carb surprises are listed also:

Corned Beef	6 oz.	0.8
Calf Liver	6 oz.	8.8
Bacon	3 slices	1.0
Spam	2 oz.	1.7
Frankfurter	1 frank	2.0
Chorizo	2 oz.	1.1
Baked deli ham	6 oz.	3.2
Honey cured deli ham	6 oz.	3.8
Pancetta	-	0.0
Beef pastrami	1 slice	0.6
Pepperoni	-	0.0
Prosciutto	-	0.0
Sliced roast beef	2 oz.	6.0
Beef and pork salami	3 slices	1.0
Clams	2 oz.	2.9
Steamed lobster	6 oz.	1.5
Steamed mussels	2 oz.	4.2
Fried octopus	4 oz.	3.3
Shelled oysters	2 oz.	6.2
Scallops	1 scallop	1.0
Cooked peeled shrimps	6 oz.	2.6
Steamed squid	6 oz.	6.4
Chicken liver	4 oz.	1.3
Turkey bacon	2 oz.	1.8
Turkey sausage	2 oz.	1.5

Meatballs	1 meatball	1.2
Seitan	2 oz.	7.0
Tempeh	2 oz.	2.5
Firm tofu	2 oz.	1.2
Soft tofu	2 oz.	1.6

Vegetables

It's important to include vegetables in your diet for the additional vitamins and mineral that they provide, as well as fiber to help digest food. Green leafy vegetables and salad are the best things to go for when planning your diet as they are still relatively low in carbohydrates, especially those high in fiber, as this can be taken away to leave a pretty small number of net grams of carbs. Starchy vegetables are best to avoid as these will take up a lot of your net carbohydrate allowance for the day. However, avocado is a great choice as it provides a high fat content as well as being pretty low in net carbs. The listings below are raw unless specified otherwise:

Steamed artichoke	1	4.0
Arugula	1 cup	0.4
Steamed asparagus	6 stems	1.9
Hass avocado	1	2.6
Steamed green beans	1 cup	5.8
Steamed pak choy	1 cup	0.8
Steamed broccoli	1 cup	3.6
Steamed cauliflower	1 cup	3.4
Steamed Brussel sprouts	1 cup	7.0
Steamed shredded cabbage	1 cup	5.4

Shredded cabbage	1 cup	2.2
Celery	1 stalk	1.0
Steamed celeriac	1 cup	7.2
Sliced cucumber	1 cup	3.2
Whole cucumber	1	9.4
Cooked eggplant	1 cup	4.6
Minced garlic	2 tablespoons	5.3
Garlic	1 clove	1.0
Steamed kale	1 cup	4.8
Cooked leeks	4 oz.	7.5
Iceberg lettuce	1 cup	1.3
Cooked button mushrooms	1 cup	9.6
Cooked shitake mushrooms	1 cup	4.0
Canned black olives	5 olives	0.7
Canned green olives	5 olives	0.1
Cooked chopped onions	1 cup	17.2
Cooked chopped bell pepper	1 cup	6.4
Chopped green bell pepper	1 cup	4.4
Jalapeno chilies	1 chili	0.5
Cooked mashed pumpkin	1 cup	9.4
Spring onions/scallions	1 cup	4.8
Cooked spring onions	1 cup	11.0
Cooked squash	1 cup	5.2
Alfalfa beansprouts	1 cup	0.1
Mung beansprouts	1 cup	4.4
Steamed sliced zucchini	1 cup	3.0
Cherry tomatoes	10	4.6
Cooked tomatoes	1 cup	17.2
Steamed mashed turnips	1 cup	7.0
Steamed sliced beetroot	1 cup	13.6
Carrots	1	4.1
Steamed sliced carrots	1 cup	8.2
Corn on the cob	1	19.6

Canned sweetcorn	1 cup	29.8
Steamed sliced parsnips	1 cup	20.4
Fresh peas	1 cup	13.8
Baked potato with skin	1	26.2
Steamed mashed potato	1 cup	30.4
Baked sweet potato	1	19.8
Mashed sweet potato	1 cup	34.8

Legumes

Beans, lentils and chick peas are a great addition to your keto diet plan as they add some extra protein and fiber. The net grams of carbohydrates will add up quickly though so it's best to add in small quantities. A couple of tablespoons of beans or lentils are a good choice to bulk up soups and stews and shelled edamame beans with a little salt are a great low carbohydrate and super healthy snack. All the listed items are cooked/canned:

Black beans 3.3	2 tablespoons
Black-eyed peas 3.1	2 tablespoons
Butter beans 3.3	2 tablespoons
Cannellini beans 3.5	2 tablespoons
Chick peas/Garbanzos 5.5	2 tablespoons
Kidney beans 3.0	2 tablespoons
Lentils	2 tablespoons

2.0	
Lima beans	2 tablespoons
3.1	
Navy beans	2 tablespoons
5.1	
Split peas	2 tablespoons
3.2	
Pinto beans	2 tablespoons
3.2	
Shelled edamame (soy)	1 cup
6.0	

Fruits

For those with a sweet tooth, the keto diet can seem like rather a challenge. However, those who follow the diet carefully usually find their cravings for sweet foods completely disappear. It's still nice to have a little fruit now and then but as you'll see from the listings below; the keto diet and fruit don't really mix. However, there are a few things you can still enjoy, for instance simply adding a few blackberries or raspberries on your plate for breakfast or a snack can be a nice sweet treat that's healthy too! And rhubarb is a real winner; pretty much the fruit with the lowest grams of net carbs. It can be really tasty when stewed with a little sweetener and served with thick cream. All the fruits listed are fresh and raw unless otherwise specified:

Apples	1
26	

Apricots	1	
3.2		
Bananas	1	
20.4		
Blackberries	1 cup	
6.6		
Blueberries	1 cup	
18.0		
Cherries	1 cup	
21.4		
Shredded coconut	1 cup	
5.0		
Cranberries	1 cup	
7.6		
Currants	1 cup	
10.6		
Dates	1	
5.3		
Figs	1	
6.5		
Gooseberries	1 cup	
7.8		
Grapefruit	1	
17.8		
Grapes	1 cup	
26.0		
Kiwi	1	
8.1		
Lychee		1
1.5		
Mango	1 cup	
22.2		
Honeydew melon	1 cup	

14.4		
Watermelon	1 cup	
11.0		
Nectarines	1	
12.6		
Oranges	1	
13.0		
Papayas	1 cup	
13.2		
Peaches	1	
10.5		
Pears	1	
20.0		
Pineapple	1 cup	
19.6		
Plums	1	
6.6		
Raspberries	1 cup	
6.8		
Strawberries	1 cup	
9.6		
Dried apricots	6 halves	
11.6		
Dried cranberries	2 tablespoons	
5.8		
Dried currants	2 tablespoons	
12.1		
Raisins	2 tablespoons	
13.6		
Dried dates	1 oz.	
20.9		
Dried figs	1	
4.5		

Rhubarb	1 cup
3.4	

Nuts and Seeds

Packed full of all the good kinds of fats, nuts and seeds make great snacks or additions to other dishes, for example salads, to boost both the flavor and the nutritional value of a dish. Obviously if you're allergic to any kinds of nuts you should make sure to omit them from your diet, however but many people are just allergic to one kind or another so it might be possible to say, add walnuts but not peanuts to your salads. Nuts and seeds are extremely versatile and can also be made into milks, flours and oils. The list below shows several different net carb ratings for reasonable portion sizes for each:

Almonds	6
0.7	
Brazil nuts	6
1.4	
Cashew nuts	2 tablespoons
7.6	
Chia seeds	2 tablespoons
1.3	
Flaxseeds	2 tablespoons
1.3	
Hazelnuts	2 tablespoons
2.4	
Hemp seeds	2 tablespoons
3.3	

Macadamia nuts	6
0.8	
Peanuts	2 tablespoons
1.4	
Pecans	10
0.6	
Pine nuts	2 tablespoons
1.6	
Shelled pistachios	2 tablespoons
3.0	
Pumpkin seeds	2 tablespoons
0.8	
Sesame seeds	2 tablespoons
2.1	
Sunflower seeds	2 tablespoons
2.0	
Walnuts	6
1.7	

Bread, Rice, Pasta, Cereals and Grains

These are all the things that you'll typically want to avoid on the keto diet, meaning it's great for anyone who's intolerant to gluten. The list is mainly here just to see how much it's possible to overload with carbs with just small quantities of these foods. However, if you're in a huge rush one morning and grab a slice of toast or half a muffin, all is not lost and you can still keep on track with your net carbs by making sure the rest of the day you eat only foods with extremely low values of net carbohydrates. The general consensus however is that it's not worth wasting so much of your daily allowance on these kinds of foods when you could be eating a much larger (and healthier) portion of vegetables instead. A small snack of popcorn is a fairly low net carb snack and using almond flour to bake instead of regular flour makes a huge different to the amount of net carbs. All listings are in reasonable serving sizes:

White bread	1 slice	
12.1		
Brown bread	1 slice	
9.8		
White pitta	1 pitta	
32.1		
Brown pitta	1 pitta	
30.5		
Flour tortilla	1	tortilla
14.5		
Corn tortilla	1	tortilla
10.8		
English muffin	1	muffin
12.0		
Cornflakes	1 cup	
11.7		
Rolled cooked oats	1 cup	
24.1		
Bran cereal	1 cup	
26.0		
Puffed rice	1 cup	
12.0		
Puffed wheat	1 cup	
10.0		
Homemade popcorn	1 cup	

5.3	
Cooked egg noodles	1 cup
38.4	
Cooked rice noodles	1 cup
42.0	
Cooked spaghetti	1 cup
30.8	
Cooked macaroni	1 cup
40.6	
Cooked white rice	1 cup
43.8	
Cooked basmati rice	1 cup
48.0	
Cooked quinoa	1 cup
34.4	
Cooked couscous	1 cup
34.2	
Cooked bulgur wheat	1 cup
25.6	
Cooked pearl barley	1 cup
38.4	
White flour	1 cup
92	
Whole wheat flour	1 cup
74	
Oat flour	1 cup
48	
Rice flour	1 cup
116	
Cornmeal	1 cup
77.6	
Almond flour	1 cup
12	

Dairy Products and Non-Dairy Alternatives

Cheese is a great way to add to the fat content of your diet in a delicious low carb way, however it's important to check the packaging as most cheese has a small amount of carbohydrates present and this varies quite a lot between varieties. Cheese and cream are so versatile and can easily be added to many dishes, or even served simply with a small number of berries or olives, for instance. Remember to always go for the highest fat content available; you definitely don't want to go for low fat options which often have added sugars. The non-dairy milk alternatives are unsweetened options; sweetened will obviously be higher in grams of net carbs. If you're not keen on having cream in your coffee or tea then almond milk can be a great alternative in trying to keep those net carbs down. Everything is listed in typical serving sizes for each item:

American sliced cheese	1 slice	
1.5		
Crumbled blue cheese	2 tablespoons	
0.4		
Brie	1 oz.	
0.1		
Camembert	1 oz.	
0.1		
Cheddar	1 oz.	
0.4		
Cottage cheese	1 cup	

	12.0	
Cream cheese		2 tablespoons
	2.0	
Edam		1 oz.
	0.4	
Feta		1 oz.
	1.2	
Goat's cheese		1 oz.
	0.3	
Monterey		1 oz.
	0.2	
Mozzarella		1 oz.
	0.6	
Grated parmesan		2 tablespoons
	0.4	
Ricotta		2 tablespoons
	1.0	
Swiss cheese		1 oz.
	1.5	
Ghee (clarified butter)		1 tablespoon
	0.0	
Butter		1 cup
	0.1	
Margarine		1 cup
	1.6	
Condensed milk		1 tablespoon
	20.8	
Thick cream		1 tablespoon
	0.4	
Soured cream		2 tablespoons
	0.7	
Whole milk		1 cup
	7.3	

Almond milk	1 cup	
1.0		
Rice milk	1 cup	
25.0		
Soy milk	1 cup	
10.0		
Coconut milk	1 cup	
6.4		
Yogurt	4 oz.	
5.3		

Condiments, Sauces and Cooking Ingredients

It's usually not necessary to pay too much attention to the odd sprinkle of black pepper or herbs but if you're using more than a dash then you'll want to log the carbs as it's surprising how quickly they can add up. Sauces and condiments make all the difference to the taste of a dish but seeing as they vary a lot in terms of carbs, it's good to know which ones to keep in the pantry. Eggs feature in this list too and being high in fat and protein and very low in carbs, they feature in many a breakfast recipe for those in ketosis. Most oils are also completely carb free so they are a great option for cooking, adding to salads, and also boosting fat content for the day.

Eggs	1 medium	
0.4		
Oil	-	
0.0		
Cocoa powder	2 tablespoons	

2.7
| Ground cinnamon | 1 teaspoon |

0.7
| Cream of tartar | 1 teaspoon |

1.8
| Flaxseed meal | 2 tablespoons |

1.0
| Molasses | 2 tablespoons |

30.0
| White sugar | 1 teaspoon |

4.2
| Pure vanilla extract | - |

0.0
| Ground nutmeg | 1 teaspoon |

0.6
| Ground allspice | 1 teaspoon |

1.0
| Dried basil | 1 tablespoon |

0.2
| Dried bay leaves | I leaf |

0.1
| Drained capers | 1 tablespoon |

0.2
| Celery salt | - |

0.0
| Chili powder | 1 tablespoon |

0.1
| Chinese 5 spice powder | 1 tablespoon |

0.1
| Dried chopped chives | 1 tablespoon |

0.1
| Ground cloves | 1 teaspoon |

0.1

Ground coriander 0.1	1 tablespoon
Ground cumin 0.1	1 teaspoon
Curry powder 0.1	1 tablespoon
Garlic powder 1.6	1 teaspoon
Ground ginger 3.1	1 tablespoon
Dried oregano 0.8	1 tablespoon
Ground paprika 1.3	1 tablespoon
Ground black pepper 4.0	1 tablespoon
Dried rosemary 0.8	1 tablespoon
Ground sage 0.1	1 teaspoon
Dried thyme 0.8	1 tablespoon
Italian seasoning 0.1	1 tablespoon
Fresh grated ginger 1.0	1 tablespoon
Fresh chopped parsley 0.2	1 tablespoon
Fresh chopped basil 0.1	1 tablespoon
Fresh chopped cilantro 0.1	2 tablespoons
Miso paste	1 tablespoon

3.0	
Honey mustard	1 teaspoon
1.0	
Dijon mustard	1 teaspoon
1.0	
Spicy brown mustard	1 teaspoon
0.1	
Peanut butter	2 tablespoons
4.0	
Tomato puree	2 tablespoons
2.2	
Worcestershire sauce	1 teaspoon
1.0	
Tahini	2 tablespoons
5.0	
Wasabi paste	1 teaspoon
2.0	
Balsamic vinegar	1 tablespoon
2.7	
Cider vinegar	1 tablespoon
0.1	
Rice vinegar	1 tablespoon
0.1	
White wine vinegar	1 tablespoon
1.5	
Barbecue sauce	1 tablespoon
1.5	
Cranberry sauce	1 tablespoon
6.5	
Apple sauce	1 tablespoon
6.0	
Ketchup	1 tablespoon
2.0	

Mayonnaise	1 tablespoon	
0.1		
Pesto	1 tablespoon	
0.6		
Soy sauce	1 tablespoon	
1.2		
Beef broth	1 cube	
0.6		
Chicken broth	1 cube	
1.1		
Vegetable broth	1 cube	
1.1		

Drinks

The nature of the keto diet is that especially in the beginning you may find you get easily dehydrated. Therefore, it's really important to keep your fluid intake up. Water is the best beverage in terms of health and zero carbs, so try and keep a bottle filled up near you at all times to encourage you to drink. You can also indulge in tea and coffee, diet soda and even the odd tipple. Drinking alcohol, however, can mess with your ketosis, even when drinking spirits which have zero grams of net carbs. You should check your ketone levels the next morning to see whether your body allows you to drink alcohol and still stay in ketosis. Fruit juices and non-diet sodas should be avoided at all costs, unless you are just using a very small amount for cooking. The following is a short list of drinks, alcoholic and non-alcoholic with net carb amounts for typical serving sizes:

Soda   12 oz.
          35.2
Diet soda   -
          0.0
Lime juice   2 tablespoons
          2.4
Lemon juice   2 tablespoons
          2.0
Apple juice   4 oz.
          13.8
Grapefruit juice   4 oz.
          13.8
Fresh orange juice   4 oz.
          12.7
Black tea   -
          0.0
Black coffee   -
          0.0
Light beer   12 oz.
          5.6
Champagne   2 oz.
          2.5
White wine   4 oz.
          2.5
Red wine   4 oz.
          3.1

days. It's far more economically friendly to buy a large block of cheese, than buy small packets of individually wrapped and sliced, or bags of pre-grated, not to mention better for the environment. Cheese that comes already grated is also sometimes dusted with corn flour so it's not only lazy but may also be higher in carbs.

Buy Smart

Sometimes it's ok to scrimp on quality and sometimes it's not. Knowing what to spend your money on is really important and will help both your bank balance and your waistline. Here are a few examples of when to scrimp and when to spend:

Ground Beef – It's fine to go for the cheaper fattier options with a higher percentage of fat. It can help you reach your nutrition targets when it comes to fat percentage, and you can even pour some of it into a container and keep in the fridge to use as cooking lard.

Oils – It's important to go for some quality oils but if you don't want to splash out on loads of different ones then just go for a decent olive oil and coconut oil. Both can be used for cooking and salads, and coconut oil is good for baking as well.

Bacon – Bacon is such a versatile food item on the keto diet but you don't need to splash out on the most expensive kinds. Again, with the more expensive items, you are usually paying to have the leaner cuts, but with the keto diet that's not what you're after! Stock up on bacon and use it to flavor soups, to wrap around asparagus spears for a snack, or just with your eggs in the morning.

Eggs – The slightly more expensive free-range or organic eggs are usually a lot tastier, and ethically better than the cheap varieties where the poor chickens have barely had room to move. And if you bulk buy you are likely to get a good price. Because eggs are such a staple of the keto diet, you should buy the best quality you can afford and you could even find out if there's a farm near you that sells them.

Sausages – Cheaper sausages are more likely to have extra fillers and therefore carbohydrates added. But if the packaging says otherwise then there's no reason not to use them on occasion.

Smart Swaps

If a recipe calls for an expensive item, you can usually find a cheaper alternative. For instance, instead of steak, go for a cheaper cut, or ground beef. If it's supposed to be a casserole made with chicken breasts, consider throwing in chicken thighs instead. IF a recipe calls for fish, maybe opt for the canned variety instead.

When it comes to vegetables, as well as avoiding fancy packaged ones, it's easier to go for the cheaper varieties. As well as being really low in carbohydrates, broccoli and cauliflower are some of the cheapest vegetables to buy. There's no need to buy bok choy and asparagus for every meal when there are much cheaper options out there. Zucchinis, lettuce, carrots and spinach are all good low-cost and fairly low-carb vegetable options.

Cheese can also be pricey but again, if the recipe says you should put an expensive brand in, just swap it out for something you can afford (checking the carbs of course). Don't be afraid to mix things up and try different things.

Chapter 9: Exercise in Ketosis – The Essentials to Know

To change your body shape and lose weight, the most important thing is diet. Therefore, exercise is not necessary while on the keto diet in order to continue losing weight. But everyone knows that exercise is good for the body, and if you were exercising before you'll likely want to continue, for the health benefits as well as feeling good about yourself.

Exercising while your body is in a state of ketosis is a little different because of the lack of carbohydrates in your body. Your body will behave differently because there are no carbohydrates to burn and therefore muscles won't be able to function for very long at all at high intensity.

Keeping a close check on your ratio of carbs, proteins and fats is very important when adding exercise to your ketogenic lifestyle, and especially the amount of protein we consume. Protein is a really useful to our bodies for many reasons. It keeps us feeling full and satisfied for longer and it also has a higher calorie burning effect. Without it we would start to lose muscle mass and also get hungry, causing us to eat more calories and put on weight.

The recommended amount of protein for athletes is between 0.6 and 0.9 grams per pound of body weight per day. You could even up that, if you are extremely active and also want to lose weight, to between 1 and 1.3 grams per pound of body weight. For someone weighing 200 pounds that would mean eating upwards of 120 grams of protein a day. This is the equivalent of around 20 eggs or 5 chicken breasts.

The best sources of protein when on the keto diet are without a doubt meat fish and eggs. Some high-fat dairy sources can also add grams of protein and you might even want to start drinking low-carb protein shakes.

When it comes to exercise on the keto diet, it really depends on how serious of an athlete you are. For those who do a lot of weight training or high intensity interval training, a very specialized nutritional plan is advised, catered to the exact requirements of the individual.

However, for those who just want to keep active, the keto diet works best with low and moderate intensity workouts, including cardio and light weight training. It's advised to get your heart rate up to between 50% to 70% of your maximum. This can generally be calculated by taking away your age from 220 to find out your estimated maximum heart rate, and then work out what 50% and 70% of this is. Therefore, someone who's 40 years old would want to be working out at a heart rate of between 90 and 126 beats per minute.

The kind of exercise you do is up to you, but anything from running, to swimming, to cycling is possible, as well as playing recreational sports such as baseball or kickball. You'll have to remember that because of being in ketosis, you might find your power and strength in some of these activities decreases but as long as you're keeping your heart rate up you'll still be achieving the health benefits.

The benefits of endurance training, or cardio, include increasing muscle mass as well as improving your coordination and balance. It also increases your bone density which is great to fend off osteoporosis and help prevent breaking or fracturing bones. Endurance training also enhances your immune system because it creates extra proteins in the body which produce antibodies and white blood cells. After training for a while you'll also notice that your body recovers much more quickly and you don't suffer so much from the aching that you often get after exercising.

The more muscle we have in our bodies, the faster we become at metabolizing calories. Our metabolism naturally decreases as we grow older so this is especially important when reaching middle age.

Exercise is also important for keeping our brains and hearts healthy. It increases blood circulation, transporting oxygen faster to our brain, and also helps to focus and release stress. Side effects include being able to get to sleep faster, sleeping better, and therefore feeling more refreshed upon waking in the morning.

There are numerous benefits to exercising and including 30 minutes to an hour of cardio a few times a week is an excellent way to supplement the good you are already doing by following the keto   diet.

Chapter 10: What about Intermittent Fasting?

You've probably heard the term intermittent fasting, or IF before. It's becoming really popular, and not just when it comes to the keto diet but in regard to other eating and training plans too.

When it comes to IF and the keto diet, it's really down to each individual and whether they want to do it or not. It can be a great way to kick start weight loss again after a bit of a plateau, and is also a lot easy when it comes to food planning and preparation. It certainly doesn't suit everyone but this chapter should tell you enough about it to decide whether it's right for you or not. As with anything, if you are planning on drastically changing your lifestyle, it's a good idea to tell your doctor first.

So, what is intermittent fasting? Well, we all know what fasting is, so it doesn't take a rocket scientist to work out that IF means fasting in small doses. How much or little time you fast for is up to you, but most people will either skip one or two mealtimes, or only eat during a specific window of time. Some people even fast for up to three days at a time, however obviously this is only occasional.

Most people find that fasting for between 18 to 20 hours a day works well and even though that may sound daunting, remember that the time you're sleeping is included in this. It gives you a 6 or 4 hour window to eat all of your calories for the day.

If you're wondering why anyone would want to put themselves through such torture, then maybe it's best to look at all the benefits associated, as losing weight is just one of them.

Losing Weight

As already mentioned, using IF can really boost your weight-loss potential. When we fast, we are basically putting our bodies into ketosis, just like what we are doing while feeding too. Seeing as we are already in a state of ketosis, it makes it really easy for our bodies to stay that way and to use stored fat in our body for fuel, just like normal.

Even though the keto diet encourages snacking on allowed foods whenever feeling hungry, it is still possible to overeat. Many people reach for the snacks because they confuse boredom with hunger so IF is great for those with tendencies to overeat. It's very difficult to overeat when you only have a few hours to eat your entire amount of food for the day.

Tracking Nutrients

When you're eating all your food in a small window of time, it's easy to remember everything you've eaten and track it accurately. One of the biggest problems for those following the keto diet is forgetting how many snacks they had and not adding them to their total carb count for the day. When you only have 4 hours to think about, it's hard to miss anything.

Mental Focus

When we're not distracting our bodies with an intake of calories throughout the day, our minds become a lot more focused. You may worry that you'll feel hungry but being on the keto diet will actually help with this. Your body is already in ketosis, so fasting just means our liver keeps producing ketones and everything ticks along as usual, with your body burning fat for fuel and providing a consistent energy source.

Physical Performance

These days everyone seems to have some special pre- or post- workout meal or shake that aids their performance and or/recovery. However, studies have shown that your performance can actually increase when you train during a fasting period. And far from negatively effecting muscle gains, fasting has even been shown to improve them. When you finally eat after fasting and training, your body will even absorb nutrients faster, leading to better results.

Autophagy

This is the process of damaged cells digesting themselves. It may sound a bit worrying but recent reports have shown that this process is actually very good for our bodies. However, if we are constantly providing our bodies with protein and fat, there is not much time for this to take place. When we rid our body of needing to process the food that we eat, it can concentrate on some maintenance work instead, and get rid of damaged cells that are not helping us to work out and could even turn cancerous.

Autophagy can be compared to our body spring-cleaning itself. And intermittent fasting paired with maintaining a constant state of ketosis even when eating, can increase the effect of autophagy.

Convenience

Preparing and cooking three or four meals a day is time consuming, even when it's simple meals. Intermittent fasting means that you can wait until you're home at night and then have a huge feast. It's a lot easier and a lot less time consuming.

Whether you choose to implement intermittent fasting or not to your lifestyle is completely up to you. You shouldn't worry that if you don't you're not going to lose weight; eating at regular times of the day while in ketosis will still have a great loss effect and you should only consider intermittent fasting if it will be convenient for you.

Chapter 11: Supplements on the Keto Diet

Many people find that they can follow the ketogenic diet without needed to take any additional pills, supplements or powders. However, to do this you must be really careful to get all the vitamins and minerals your body needs each day. Our bodies are clever and adaptable and it might take a while to know whether we're missing out on any of the micronutrients that we need to function. Therefore, it can be wise to consider taking a number of supplements to ensure you stay fit and healthy and your body gets everything it needs.

When embarking on your keto journey you don't want any deficiencies to get in the way of your weight loss success, and certainly not your health. So, if you can afford to, at the very least, get some multivitamins, you can be sure your body isn't missing out and you can concentrate fully on maintaining a state of ketosis.

Multivitamin tablet – Generic vitamin and mineral tablet, some aimed specifically towards gender.

Vitamin D tablet – Busy schedules mean that a lot of people just don't get enough time in the sun and that's the only way our bodies can produce vitamin D, deficiencies of which have been linked to strokes, heart disease, diabetes and osteoporosis.

Magnesium – This is also a natural muscle relaxant so it's great to take before bed, and out of all the different magnesiums available, magnesium citrate is the form that absorbs most easily into the body.

Fish Oil – Even with the vast amounts of meat and eggs eaten on the keto diet, it's good to make sure you're getting enough of the right kind of Omega 3-fatty acids and if you're not eating much fish this would be a good supplement to take.

Melatonin – Studies have shown that a deprivation of sleep can cause people to overeat and consume up to 45% more calories so to make sure you get as good night's sleep, supplementing with melatonin is a good choice.

MCT Oil – Great for adding extra fat to your diet, this oil is absorbed really quickly so it's a great boost for your body producing more ketones in the liver.

Specialized Keto Supplements – There are many products that are specifically created for those following the keto diet, including pre- and post workout protein shakes, as well as nutritional supplements, such as Perfect Keto and KetoShred.

Chapter 12: Advanced Tips for Staying in Ketosis

We all need keeping in check at times, and while following any new lifestyle change it takes time and it's a challenge sometimes. When you do things many times however, they slowly become routine, and then just a habit that we do without thinking. However, even when things become a habit, we can become sloppy, so below are a few reminders about how to keep on track as well as what to do when eating out and some other advanced tips.

Weighing Yourself

Although it might be tempting to weigh yourself every day, it can actually be better to stick to a weekly weigh in. Everyone's weight fluctuates to some extent and getting bogged down with minor increases and decreases from one day to the next can be distracting and demotivating. Pick one day a week, in the morning on an empty stomach and make a note of it in your keto diary or journal. It's much more satisfying to see yourself losing steadily over the weeks rather than half a pound here and there from one day to the next.

Eating Out

Although it's best to keep eating out to a minimum

as it's harder to track your net carbs, there are going to be social occasions where you will want to be able to enjoy food with your friends and family. Whether it's going to a restaurant or eating at someone's house, there are a few ways to ensure you don't fall off the keto wagon. Brunch is a great meal to suggest going out for as you can opt for something egg-based such as an omelet or poached eggs with spinach and salmon.

Restaurants – Ask if there are any low-carb options or adapt one of the menu options to suit a keto meal. In Indian and Chinese restaurants, the rice is usually ordered separately so you can go for a meat-based savory dish and skip the rice/naan/prawn crackers. In burger joints, just leave the bun or ask for it to be swapped out for a little salad. Most meals can be adapted in some way in order to make more keto-friendly and don't be afraid of asking the waiting staff to change your dish.

Dinner at someone's house – It can be awkward turning up at someone's house when you're on a diet and don't know what will be for dinner. Calling up beforehand and explaining how important it is that you don't eat too many carbs is a great way to pre-warn people. There's nothing worse than getting to dinner and then having to pick around your plate and not be able to eat anything. It's awkward for you, and it's rude to your host. By giving some tips beforehand about what you can eat, and asking to skip any high carb sides, you can still enjoy a nice evening out, and without going hungry.

Barbecues – Great for those on the keto diet, barbecues are easy to just select the meat option, just don't be tempted by too many sides. Because they're usually very relaxed and social events, you can usually even bring your own meat if you're worried about any sweet marinades other people may have added. A burger or piece of chicken with some cheese and a small amount of salad is a perfect keto meal.

Water!

Water, water, water. It's vital for life and when you're dehydrated will cause you to feel tired, unfocused and even depressed. Because of the nature of the keto diet it's important to up your water intake and an easy way to do this is to get into the habit of drinking a large glass of water as soon as you wake up in the morning, before every meal, and also before going to bed at night. Carrying around a water bottle will help you remember to drink and is also more eco-friendly than buying bottles of water all the time. Drinking before mealtimes will also help with not overrating, which leads on to the next advanced tip.

Overeating

One of the great things about the keto diet is that

there are some things you can eat unlimited quantities of. However, this shouldn't be an excuse to gorge on meats and cheeses out of boredom. It's a good idea to have snacks prepared for when you're feeling a bit peckish in between meals, but eating a whole roast chicken late at night after you've already eaten three or four meals is not a good habit to get into. Drinking plenty of water will fill up your stomach, keep you hydrated, and also help prevent overeating.

Eating Too Many Carbohydrates

Linked to overeating, letting your net carb creep up during the day by indulging in extra snacks is going to take you out of ketosis and affect your weight loss journey, especially if you are eating a lot of cheese and eggs as snacks and aren't adding the net carbs to your keto diary. Even though there are such a small amount of carbohydrates in cheese and eggs, it's still really important to count everything; it all adds up. Also, be careful on meats, because deli meats especially often have added ingredients and if you're snacking on them assuming they're zero carbs, it could kick you out of ketosis.

Another way to make sure you're not eating too many carbohydrates is to make sure you're a stickler for weighing out food before you cook it. Being sloppy about portion sizes and guessing can add enough net carbs to affect the progress of your weight loss.

Eating Too Little Carbohydrates

Even though the ketogenic diet is all about restricting carbohydrate intake, it's really important to make sure you still get enough of them. It's easy to concentrate on the foods you can eat plenty of and forget about your 25 or 30 grams of carbs. However, not getting enough carbohydrates can be dangerous as well as just unhealthy. We need carbohydrates for healthy brain function (even though the brain mostly prefers fats) and we also need all the vitamins and nutrients that vegetables provide.

Test Your Ketones

The only way to truly know if you are in ketosis, and have the right amount of ketones in your bloodstream is to test for it. You can do this by picking up some tests from a pharmacy or drug store. There are urine strips where you simply pee on the strip, or blood tests where you have to prick yourself to get a reading. The latter are usually more accurate but either are recommended in order to check that you're in ketosis in the first place, and then to check that your ketone level isn't too high. The ideal range that you are looking for is somewhere between 0.5 mol/L and 3.0 mol/L.

Supplements

In order to get all the vitamins, minerals and nutrients that your body needs, it's a good idea to consider taking supplements, even if you're not working out frequently. It's also a good idea to mix up taking different supplements; try different brands or different varieties of nutrients. You'll learn what works for you and makes you feel the best.

Mix Things Up!

Don't let boredom cause you to become demotivated and start eating unsuitable foods and drinks. The keto diet is great, because you can keep it really simple so that's it's easy to weigh out quantities of only a small amount of ingredients for easy carb tracking and convenience. However, make the effort to try some new dishes when you have a little extra time and it'll make all the difference and keep you from getting in a rut. Changing up which vegetables you use will provide your body with different kinds of nutrients, and adding spices have great additional benefits, for instance turmeric for its inflammatory properties, and ginger which can be great for settling the stomach.

If you struggle to get time to cook in the evenings, try cooking in bulk during the weekends, so that you have the time to try out new recipes, and can also stock up on good healthy and tasty keto meals for during the week.

Weight Loss Plateaus

On every diet there comes a time when you seem to get stuck and your weight doesn't seem to budge. This may be the time to take a look at your net carbs and possibly think about decreasing the amount slightly. You should also evaluate whether you are drinking enough water, and whether you are overeating.

Chapter 13: Keto Meal Plan with Recipes

This food plan has been put together specifically for this book and delivers an overall meal plan for each day consisting of around 2000 calories with a ratio of 5 to 10% net carbs, 70 to 75% fat and 20 to 25% protein. It centers around wholefoods and recipes and snacks which are really easy to put together. Some of the meals can be cooked in batches when they are suitable to be used as leftover meals. There is a close eye to detail to make sure this keto diet plan includes as many as your recommended daily vitamins, minerals and nutrients. However, please refer to the chapter on supplements if you would prefer to take a vitamin supplement as well.

The number of grams of net carbs are clearly stated at the end of each recipe. Some of the recipes have been repeated to show example of how to plan, batch cook, and enjoy again the next day. This is a great idea for lunches, especially if you're going to be at work or school. If they provide a microwave you can easily heat up leftover meals, or else make things that are good to eat cold.

The recipes that follow are ordered in a typical breakfast, lunch, dinner and a snack format. However, you can just mix and match the recipes to suit your needs and what you fancy. If you've chosen to include intermittent fasting to your diet then your breakfast might be a lot later in the day, when you might choose to have a salad instead of something breakfasty. But breakfast-type meals (eggs, bacon, sausage, etc.) are also a great choice for dinner. You just need to keep an eye on the carb ratings for each meal and make sure that your daily allowance doesn't get too high (over around 25g of net carbs).

With the help of a carb counter – either from this book or from your own calorie counter book or app, you can adapt each recipe to suit yourself. Don't like Brussel sprouts or cabbage? Simply switch in another vegetable for the same amount of net carbs. Meats are even easier to swap as you don't even need to take into account carbs.

Day One

Breakfast:
Cheese and Chive Omelet

Ingredients:
3 eggs
1oz. grated Monterey cheese
½ tablespoon fresh chopped chives
1 tablespoon thick cream
¼ avocado

Instructions:
Crack the eggs into a bowl and beat with a fork.
Add the thick cream, chopped chives and a pinch
of salt to the mixture.
Pour into a hot pan and let cook, sprinkle over the
grated cheese.
When the bottom side is cooked, flip and cook the
other side.
Serve with another sprinkling of grated cheese and
chopped chives.
Slice the avocado and arrange on top.

The net carb rating for this dish is **2.6 grams**.

Lunch:
Hummus and Olive Salad

Ingredients:
1 tablespoon hummus
1 tablespoon olive oil

4 cups shredded lettuce
1 grated carrot
½ cup chopped green olives
2 eggs

Instructions:
Boil the eggs for 6 minutes and put to the side to cool.
Mix the shredded lettuce, grated carrot and chopped olives, and arrange on a plate.
Peel the eggs and slice them, arranging over the salad.
Finish with a dollop of hummus and a drizzle of olive oil.

The net carb rating for this dish is **9.6 grams**.

Dinner:
Meaty Low Carb Pizza (Makes 4 servings)

Ingredients:
4 oz. grated cheddar cheese
8 oz. grated/torn mozzarella cheese
3 eggs
3 cloves minced garlic
2 tablespoons ground flaxseed
1 tablespoon Italian herbs
¼ cup tomato sauce
5 oz. pepperoni
5 oz. turkey salami
5 oz. chorizo
¼ lb. sliced mushrooms
¼ cup sliced green bell pepper

Instructions:

Mix the cheese, eggs, garlic, Italian herbs and flaxseed together and put to one side.

Preheat the oven to 450.

Line a pizza tray with parchment paper or aluminum foil and spray with cooking oil.

Spread the cheesy 'dough' as thinly as possible inside the pan.

Cook for about 10 minutes, or until golden brown.

Spread the tomato sauce over the pizza base and then top with pepperoni, salami and chorizo.

Finally top with sliced mushrooms and green pepper and any extra grated cheese.

Return to the oven for a few minutes until the toppings are satisfactorily cooked.

Use a pizza cutter to slice into 4 quarters.

The net carb rating for this dish is **7.1 grams**.

Snack:
Warm Salami Salad

Ingredients:
4 cups arugula
2 oz. turkey salami
1 tablespoon sunflower seeds
1 tablespoon grated parmesan cheese
1 tablespoon olive oil

Instructions:
Tear apart the turkey salami into smaller pieces.
Toss the arugula and turkey salami together.

Add the sunflower seeds and grated parmesan and drizzle with olive oil.

The net carb rating for this dish is **2.8 grams**.

Day Two

Breakfast:
Brussel Sprout Breakfast Hash

Ingredients:
1 tablespoon olive oil
5 rashers bacon
½ cup chopped walnuts
6 Brussel sprouts
1 egg

Instructions:
Heat the olive oil in a hot pan and add the bacon.
Fry on both sides and then put to one side.
Slice the Brussel sprouts very thinly and add to the pan.
Stir regularly but meanwhile break the bacon strips into pieces.
Add to the pan and mix together with the sprouts.
Turn pan to a very low heat and mix in walnuts.
Crack egg over hash mixture and place a lid over pan.
Cook egg to personal taste, add a little salt, and serve.

The net carb rating for this dish is **8.1 grams**.

Lunch:
Meaty Low Carb Pizza – leftovers
See Day 1 for recipe.

The net carb rating for this dish is **7.1 grams**.

Dinner:
Chicken and Zucchini Noodles

Ingredients:
1 chicken breast
½ zucchini
1 tablespoon olive oil
2 tablespoons cream cheese
2 tablespoons parmesan cheese

Instructions:
Heat oil in a pan.
Slice chicken breast into thin slices and add to pan, turning often.
Spiralize zucchini and add to pan once chicken is cooked.
Mix in cream cheese and parmesan and a sprinkle of salt.
Stir until the cheeses have melted in and serve immediately.

The net carb rating for this dish is **6.3 grams**.

Snack:
Hummus and Olives

Ingredients:
I tablespoon hummus
½ cup of olives

Instructions:

Mix together and enjoy as a snack at any time of the day.

The net carb rating for this dish is **1.6 grams**.

Day 3

Breakfast:
Cream Cheese and Green Pepper Scramble

Ingredients:
2 tablespoons olive oil
3 eggs
3 tablespoons cream cheese
½ cup chopped green bell pepper
1 teaspoon fresh chopped chives

Instructions:
Heat oil in a pan and throw in the chopped green peppers.
Stir for a few minutes.
Crack eggs one by one into the pan, stirring after each.
Finally add cream cheese and a dash of salt.
Serve with a sprinkle of chopped chives

The net carb rating for this dish is **4.1 grams**.

Lunch:
Spicy Tuna and Corn Salad

Ingredients:
2 cans tuna in spring water
2 tablespoons mayonnaise
2 tablespoons olive oil
1 diced jalapeno pepper
2 tablespoons of canned corn

Instructions:
Drain cans of tuna and add to bowl.
Pour over oil and mayonnaise and then mix in corn.
Serve with jalapeno pepper sprinkled over.

The net carb rating for this dish is **3.4 grams**.

Dinner:
Cauliflower and Chorizo 'Mac' and Cheese
(Makes 4 servings)

Ingredients:
1 whole cauliflower
1 cup thick cream
2 oz. cream cheese
2 tablespoons mustard
2 cups grated cheddar
2 cloves minced garlic
4 oz. chorizo

Instructions:
Chop the cauliflower into bite-sized florets and steam for 5 minutes.
Preheat the oven to 375 degrees.
Spray a baking tray with cooking oil.
Mix all ingredients together and pour into baking tray.
Save 1 cup of grated cheddar to sprinkle on top.
Bake for about 15 minutes or until golden brown and bubbly on top.

The net carb rating for this dish is **10.4 grams**.

Snack:
Shredded Chicken Breast 'Wraps'

Ingredients:
½ cooked shredded chicken breast
¼ cup grated Monterey cheese
2 tablespoons soured cream
5 large lettuce leaves

Instructions:
Lay out and flatten the 5 lettuce leaves.
Spread a little soured cream on each and divide up the chicken.
Sprinkle cheese on each and then roll up to form 5 lettuce wraps.

The net carb rating for this dish is **2.1 grams**.

Day 4

Breakfast:
Guacamole with Bacon (Guacamole makes 2 servings)

Ingredients:
1 avocado
1 tablespoon lime juice
1 clove minced garlic
½ diced tomato
2 tablespoons fresh chopped cilantro
1 diced spring onion
2 tablespoons olive oil
5 strips bacon

Instructions:
Mash up the avocado in a bowl.
Add all other ingredients apart from bacon and 1 tablespoon of olive oil.
Mix well with a pinch of salt.
Heat the remaining oil in a pan and fry the strips of bacon.
Serve half the guacamole with the bacon.

The net carb rating for this dish is **4.3 grams**.

Lunch:
Cauliflower and Chorizo 'Mac' and Cheese – leftovers
See Day 3 for recipe.

The net carb rating for this dish is **10.4 grams**.

Dinner:
Pan-fried Chicken Breast with Baby Spinach
(Makes 2 servings)

Ingredients:
2 chicken breasts
4 oz. brie
8 cups spinach
2 tablespoon olive oil
2 teaspoon dried sage
½ cup chopped walnuts

Instructions:
Heat the oil in a pan and add the chicken breast.
Flip after 5 minutes and top with chunks of brie
and the dried sage.
Remove from pan when cooked through and
cheese is melted.
Add baby spinach and chopped walnuts to pan and
toss in the leftover oil for a minute or two.
Serve together on a plate.

The net carb rating for this dish is **3.0 grams**.

Snack:
Guacamole with Celery

Ingredients:
Leftover guacamole from breakfast
2 celery stalks

Salmon with Garlic Sautéed Kale (Salmon makes 4 servings)

Ingredients:
12 oz. salmon in 4 pieces
1 tablespoon maple syrup
1 tablespoon hoisin sauce
1 tablespoon Dijon mustard
1 cup chopped kale
3 tablespoons olive oil
1 clove minced garlic

Instructions:
Mix together the maple syrup, hoisin sauce, mustard and 1 tablespoon of the oil in a bowl.
Preheat the oven to 375 degrees.
Lay out 4 pieces of aluminum foil and place a piece of salmon on each.
Pour even amounts of the mixture on each salmon fillet.
Turn the fillets over, making sure they are covered in the mixtures.
Wrap the foil into parcels and place on a baking tray in the oven.
Bake for about 25 minutes or until the salmon is cooked through.
Heat the rest of the oil in a pan and add the minced garlic.
Stir for a minute or two and then add the kale and fry for a few minutes.
Remove salmon from parcel and serve with the sautéed kale.

The net carb rating for this dish is **12.5 grams**.

Snack:
Mushroom 'Chips' with Sausages

Ingredients:
2 thinly sliced Portobello mushrooms
1 tablespoon ghee (clarified butter)
2oz. pork sausages

Instructions:
Preheat oven to 300 degrees.
Place mushroom slices in a single layer on a non-stick baking tray.
Brush with ghee and sprinkle with salt and pepper.
Bake for 30 mins, remove from oven and flip.
Brush with ghee and add pork sausages to the tray.
Cook for a further 20 mins or until sausages are done.
Serve together as a snack.

The net carb rating for this dish is **3.6 grams**.

Day 6

Breakfast:
Egg and Bacon Muffins

Ingredients:
1 oz. almond flour
1 egg
1 teaspoon baking soda
1 oz. grated cheddar cheese
4 slices cooked and crumbled bacon
1 tablespoon thick cream
1 tablespoon olive oil

Instructions:
Preheat oven to 375 degrees.
Mix all the ingredients together in a bowl with a little salt and pepper.
Place 4 paper muffin cases in a muffin tin and pour mixture between them.
Bake for about 20 minutes or until a knife comes out clean.
Enjoy on their own or with a little butter.

The net carb rating for this dish is **3.6 grams**.

Lunch:
Salmon Parcel – leftovers

The net carb rating for this dish is **10.2 grams**.

Dinner:

Cheesy Spinach Meatloaf (Makes 4 servings)

Ingredients:
2lbs ground beef or pork
2 eggs
3 spring onions
1 diced onion
3 cloves minced garlic
1 ½ cups spinach
4 oz. goat's cheese
2 teaspoons tomato puree
½ teaspoon cayenne pepper
½ teaspoon dried oregano
1 tablespoon fresh chopped rosemary

Instructions:
Preheat the oven to 450 degrees.
Mix together the ground meat and eggs in a bowl.
Add the spring onions, onion, garlic, tomato puree, cayenne pepper and oregano.
Pat the mixture out into a rectangle shape on a large sheet of plastic wrap.
Place the goat's cheese and spinach onto the mixture and use the plastic wrap to make a roll.
Pack tightly and leave in the fridge for ten minutes.
Spray a baking tray with cooking oil and carefully unwrap the meat loaf onto the tray.
Sprinkle with rosemary and bake for about 50 minutes until cooked through.

The net carb rating for this dish is **5.0 grams**.

Snack:

Kale Chips and Fried Eggs

Ingredients:
2 cups chopped kale
2 tablespoons olive oil
2 eggs

Instructions:
Preheat oven to 350 degrees.
Tear up kale and remove any tough stems.
Toss with olive oil and a little salt and pepper and then add to a baking tray.
Bake for 10 to 15 minutes or when the 'chips' are starting to get crispy.
Meanwhile heat up the remaining oil in a pan and add the eggs.
Serve the fried eggs on top of the crunchy kale chips.

The net carb rating for this dish is **7.7 grams**.

Day 7

Breakfast:
Eggs, Bacon and Avocado

Ingredients:
2 eggs
5 slices bacon
¼ sliced avocado
1 tablespoon olive oil

Instructions:
Heat oil in a pan and add bacon. Fry until crispy and then put to one side.
Crack eggs into pan and fry in leftover oil and bacon fat.
Serve bacon and eggs with sliced avocado on the side.

The net carb rating for this dish is **2.1 grams**.

Lunch:
Cheesy Spinach Meatloaf – leftovers
With **Roasted Brussel Sprouts**

Ingredients:
6 Brussel sprouts
1 tablespoon olive oil

Instructions:
Preheat oven to 425 degrees.
Slice sprouts into halves and toss in a pan with the

oil and a little salt and pepper.

Roast in the oven for about 25 minutes or until starting to go a little brown and crispy.

After 15 minutes of cooking, add the meatloaf to the oven to warm.

Serve the meatloaf and roasted Brussel sprouts together.

The net carb rating for this dish is **10.9 grams**.

Dinner:
Heart-warming Chicken Soup (Makes 2 servings)

Ingredients:
1 cooked shredded chicken breast
3 tablespoons butter
4 oz. cream cheese
2 cups chicken broth
½ cup thick cream
½ teaspoon garlic powder
½ teaspoon onion powder

Instructions:
Melt butter in pan and add shredded chicken, coating in butter.

Add the cream cheese, garlic and onion powder, and stir until the cream cheese melts.

Pour in the chicken broth and thick cream and stir.

Heat until it boils, then simmer for a few minutes before serving.

The net carb rating for this dish is **5.1 grams**.

Snack:
Rhubarb and Cream

Ingredients:
1 cup diced rhubarb
½ cup thick cream

Instructions:
Steam or boil the rhubarb in a small amount of water until soft.
Add a little sweetener if required.
Serve with thick cream straight from the fridge.

The net carb rating for this dish is **6.7 grams.**

Day 8

Breakfast:
Cheesy Spinach Omelet

Ingredients:
2 tablespoons butter
3 eggs
2 tablespoons grated cheddar cheese
3 cups of baby spinach leaves

Instructions:
Crack the eggs into a bowl and beat until fluffy.
Heat the butter in a pan.
Mix the cheese and egg and pour the mixture into the pan.
Turn the pan to allow the mixture to coat it.
After a couple of minutes, flip the omelet.
Add the spinach, fold in half and serve.

The net carb rating for this dish is **2.7 grams**.

Lunch:
Heart-Warming Chicken Soup – Leftovers

The net carb rating for this dish is **5.1 grams**.

Dinner:
Chili Cheeseburger (Makes 4 Servings) with
Buttery Zucchini 'Fries'

Ingredients:

2 lbs. ground beef or pork
2 diced jalapenos
4 oz. cheddar cheese
2 chicken broth cubes
1 zucchini
1 tablespoon butter
2 tablespoons grated parmesan

Instructions:
Preheat the grill to high.
Crumble the chicken broth cubes into the meat and mix in a bowl with the jalapenos.
Divide the mixture into 4 and form into patties.
Grill for about 5 minutes.
Slice the zucchinis into 'fry'-like shapes.
Heat the butter on a pan and add the 'fries' when hot, stirring often.
Turn the beef patties after 5 minutes and for the last 2 minutes add the grated cheese to the top of each burger.
When zucchini 'fries' are golden brown, serve them alongside one chili cheeseburger.

The net carb rating for this dish is **9.2 grams**.

Snack:
Smoked Salmon 'Wraps'

Ingredients:
4 oz. smoked salmon
2 tablespoons cream cheese
2 tablespoons chopped walnuts
5 large lettuce leaves

Day 10

Breakfast:
Pesto Chicken Breakfast Scramble

Ingredients:
½ cooked and shredded chicken breast
2 eggs
2 tablespoons pesto
2 tablespoons thick cream
Handful of fresh basil leaves

Instructions:
Beat eggs in a bowl with the pesto and the thick cream.
Pour into a hot non-stick pan and stir until the egg starts to cook.
Add the chicken and finish cooking.
Serve with fresh basil leaves.

The net carb rating for this dish is **3.1 grams**.

Lunch:
Brie and Walnut Salad

Ingredients:
4 slices cooked and crumbled bacon
2 oz. brie
2 cups arugula
¼ cup walnuts
1 tablespoon olive oil

Instructions:

Tear the brie into pieces and toss all ingredients together.

Can be served with warm or cold bacon.

The net carb rating for this dish is **2.5 grams**.

Dinner:
Zucchini Carbonara

Ingredients:

4 spiralized zucchinis
1 tablespoon olive oil
8 slices bacon
½ diced onion
2 cloves minced garlic
½ diced cured ham
½ cup frozen peas
3 eggs
¾ cup thick cream
¾ cup grated parmesan

Instructions:

Heat the oil in a pan and add the bacon and onion.
Stir for a few minutes until the onion starts to turn golden and add the minced garlic.
After a few more minutes add the ham, frozen peas and zucchini noodles.
Beat the eggs and stir in the cream and parmesan.
Take the pan off the heat and stir in the sauce, careful not to let the eggs scramble.
Add a dash of salt and pepper and serve warm or cold.

The net carb rating for this dish is **9.1 grams**.

Snack:
Garlic and Anchovy Hash

Ingredients:
4 oz. canned anchovies
3 cups shredded cabbage
1 clove minced garlic
1 tablespoon olive oil
3 tablespoons grated parmesan

Instructions:
Heat the oil in a pan and throw in the shredded cabbage and minced garlic.
Drain the anchovies, chop up a little and add to pan when cabbage starts to wilt a little.
Stir in the grated parmesan and serve immediately.

The net carb rating for this dish is **5.1 grams.**

ADDITIONAL RECIPES

SPECIAL NUTTY PORRIDGE

SERVES 4 PREPARATION TIME 5 MINUTES
COOKING TIME 10 MINUTES

INGREDIENTS
2 ¼ cups unsweetened almond milk
½ cup almond butter
2 tbsp. almond oil
¼ cup chia seeds
¼ cup toasted chopped pecans
¼ cup toasted chopped walnuts
¼ cup roasted sliced almond
1 tsp. cinnamon

INSTRUCTIONS

1. Pour almond milk into a pan then bring to a simmer.

2. Stir in chia seeds, pecans, walnuts, and sliced almonds, then stir well. Remove from heat.

3. Quickly add almond butter and almond oil to the pan then stir well.

4. Transfer to a serving dish then sprinkle cinnamon on top.

5. Serve and enjoy.

NUTRITION PER SERVING

CALORIES 263 PROTEIN 5.7 FIBER 5.9 SUGARS 1
FAT 24.4

TIP

This nutty porridge can be enjoyed hot or cold.
If you like, you may add cloves and nutmeg to
enhance the aroma.

ORIGINAL COCONUT PANCAKES

SERVES 4 PREPARATION TIME 8 MINUTES
COOKING TIME 10 MINUTES

INGREDIENTS

**2 organic eggs
2 tbsp. flax seeds
½ cup coconut flour
½ cup coconut milk
1 tsp. olive oil**

INSTRUCTIONS

1. Combine all ingredients in a bowl then whisk until smooth and incorporated.

2. Preheat a saucepan over medium heat then brush with olive oil.

3. Pour about 2 tablespoons of batter into the saucepan then cook for about 2 minutes.

4. Flip the pancake then cook again for another 2 minutes or until both sides of the pancake are lightly golden.

5. Repeat with the remaining batter then arrange on a serving dish.

6. Serve and enjoy.

CALORIES 136 PROTEIN 4.4 FIBER 2.2 SUGARS 1.4 FAT 11.9

TIP
Top the pancakes with fresh fruits according to your desire.

WARM SPINACH SMOOTHIE

SERVES 4 PREPARATION TIME 2 MINUTES
COOKING TIME 6 MINUTES

INGREDIENTS

**2 cups unsweetened almond milk
2 cups chopped spinach
2 medium carrots
2 tbsp. lemon juice
2 tsp. ginger**

INSTRUCTIONS

1. Peel the carrots then cut into thick slices.

2. Place the carrots in a blender then add the remaining ingredients to the blender. Process until smooth.

3. Divide the smoothie into 4 serving glasses then serve.

4. Enjoy.

NUTRITION PER SERVING

CALORIES 41 PROTEIN 1.3 FIBER 1.7 SUGARS 1.8
FAT 1.9

TIP

This smoothie is also great consumed cold. Make it
at the night before and store it in the refrigerator.

SAVORY VEGETABLE PANCAKES

SERVES 4 PREPARATION TIME 5 MINUTES
COOKING TIME 15 MINUTES

INGREDIENTS
¼ cup coconut flour
½ tsp. pepper
1 organic egg
2 tbsp. coconut milk
½ cup grated carrot
½ cup zucchini
1 cup chopped spinach
½ cup chopped onion
1 ½ tbsp. olive oil

INSTRUCTIONS

1. Combine coconut flour with pepper, egg, and coconut milk. Stir well.

2. Add carrot, zucchini, spinach, and onion then mix well.

3. Preheat a saucepan over medium heat then brush the pan with olive oil.

4. Drop about two tablespoons of batter to make the pancake. Repeat with the remaining ingredients.

5. Arrange the pancakes on a serving dish then serve immediately.

NUTRITION PER SERVING

CALORIES 98 PROTEIN 2.4 FIBER 1.5 SUGARS 2
FAT 8.3

.

LOW CARB CHEESE SANDWICH

SERVES 4 PREPARATION TIME 6 MINUTES
COOKING TIME 12 MINUTES

INGREDIENTS
8 organic eggs
½ cup mashed avocado
4 slices bacon
4 slices cheddar cheese

INSTRUCTIONS

1. Preheat a steamer then coat 8 small round baking pans with cooking spray.

2. Crack the eggs and place each egg in each baking pan.

3. Arrange the pan in the steamer then steam until the eggs are set— like making steamed sunny side up eggs.

4. Remove the baking pan from the steamer then take the steamed sunny side up eggs out of the baking pan.

5. Arrange 4 steamed eggs on a flat surface then spread mashed avocado over each egg.

6. Layer with bacon and cheese then top with the remaining steamed eggs.

7. Arrange on a serving dish then serve.

8. Enjoy.

NUTRITION PER SERVING

CALORIES 287 PROTEIN 18.6 FIBER 2 SUGARS 0.9 FAT 22.5

TIP
Make sure that you use ripe avocados for this recipe. Unripe avocados have a hard texture and bitter taste.

ZUCCHINI CUPCAKES WITH TASTY BACON

SERVES 4 PREPARATION TIME 20 MINUTES
COOKING TIME 25 MINUTES

INGREDIENTS
**2 medium zucchinis
4 slices bacon
1 cup almond flour
¼ cup chopped onion
¼ tsp. salt
½ tsp. pepper
4 organic eggs
3 tbsp. water**

INSTRUCTIONS

1. Preheat an oven to 250°F then coat 8 muffin cups with cooking spray.

2. Peel the zucchini then discard the seeds.

3. Shred the zucchini then set aside.

4. Cut the bacon into very small dice then place in the same bowl with grated zucchini.

5. Add chopped onion to the same bowl then mix well.

6. Crack the eggs then place in a separate bowl.

7. Season with salt and pepper then using an electric mixer whisk until fluffy.

8. Pour water into the beaten egg then add almond flour into it. Whisk until incorporated.

9. Add the zucchini mixture to the egg mixture and using a wooden spatula stir well.

10. Pour the mixture into the prepared muffin cups then bake for 20 minutes or until the tops of the cupcakes are lightly golden.

NUTRITION PER SERVING

CALORIES 138 PROTEIN 8.9 FIBER 2.2 SUGARS 2.6 FAT 9.6

TIP

This on-the-go breakfast can be prepared in advance so you can save time in the morning. Store this dish in a container with a lid in the refrigerator. When you want to consume, microwave on medium heat for 30 seconds then enjoy.

SALMON PLATTER

SERVES 4 PREPARATION TIME 7 MINUTES
COOKING TIME 10 MINUTES

INGREDIENTS
8 organic eggs
2 radishes
1 ripe avocado
1 tsp. olive oil
¼ tsp. salt
¼ tsp. pepper
1 cup sliced salmon

INSTRUCTIONS

1. Crack an egg then into a bowl.

2. Pour water into a saucepan then bring to a simmer.

3. Once it is simmering, gently slip the egg into the water.

4. Poach the egg until set but still soft. Repeat with the remaining eggs, cooking only one egg at a time.

5. Next, preheat a saucepan over medium heat then pour olive oil into it.

6. Once it is hot, stir in salmon fillet then season with salt and pepper.

7. Sauté until salmon is just cooked then remove from heat.

8. Divide the salmon into 4 serving dishes then add two poached eggs to each dish.

9. Peel the avocado and discard the pit. Cut the avocado flesh into small dice.

10. Place diced avocado and sliced radish on each dish then serve the salmon platter.

11. Enjoy.

NUTRITION PER SERVING

CALORIES 329 PROTEIN 22.1 FIBER 3.4 SUGARS 1 FAT 25.2

LEMON SOUFFLE WITH STRAWBERRY TOPPING

SERVES 4 PREPARATION TIME 15 MINUTES
COOKING TIME 20 MINUTES

INGREDIENTS
12 egg yolks
12 egg whites
1 ½ tsp. lemon zest
3 tbsp. lemon juice
¼ cup coconut flour
3 tsp. coconut oil
TOPPING:
1 cup fresh strawberries
½ cup water
2 tbsp. lemon juice

INSTRUCTIONS

1. First, make the topping.

2. Place fresh strawberries in a pan then pour water and lemon juice over the strawberries.

3. Bring to a simmer while stirring occasionally.

4. Remove from heat and let sit for a few minutes until thickened.

5. Meanwhile, preheat an oven to 250°F then coat a medium baking dish with cooking spray. Set aside.

6. Place egg yolks together with lemon zest, coconut flour, and coconut oil in a bowl. Whisk until incorporated.

7. In a separate bowl, place egg whites and lemon juice then whisk until foamy.

8. Stir in the egg whites to egg yolk mixture then mix until combined.

9. Pour the egg mixture into the prepared baking dish then spread evenly.

10. Drizzle strawberry topping on top then bake the casserole for approximately 20 minutes.

11. Once it is done, remove from the oven then let cool.

12. Serve and enjoy.

NUTRITION PER SERVING

CALORIES 262 PROTEIN 19.4 FIBER 1.1 SUGARS
3.2 FAT 17.5

TIP

Strawberry can be substituted with blueberry,
cranberry, raspberry, or a mix of these fruits.
Choose ripe berries, so you can enjoy the natural
sweetness.

VEGETABLE WAFFLES

SERVES 4 PREPARATION TIME 15 MINUTES
COOKING TIME 15 MINUTES

INGREDIENTS

1 cup grated carrot
4 organic eggs
¼ cup almond flour
¼ tsp. black pepper
2 tbsp. grated cheese

INSTRUCTIONS

1. Crack the eggs then combine with almond flour.

2. Season with black pepper then whisk until smooth.

3. Add grated cheese and grated carrot to the flour mixture then mix until combined.

4. Preheat a waffle maker then cook the waffles according to the machine's instructions.

5. Arrange the waffles on a serving dish then enjoy.

NUTRITION PER SERVING

CALORIES 129 PROTEIN 8.2 FIBER 1.5 SUGARS 2
FAT 9

TIP
If almond flour is too expensive, consider coconut
flour as a cheaper option.

SOFT CINNAMON PANCAKE

SERVES 4 PREPARATION TIME 4 MINUTES
COOKING TIME 15 MINUTES

INGREDIENTS
**½ cup softened cream cheese
8 organic eggs
½ cup almond yogurt
1 tsp. cinnamon**

INSTRUCTIONS

1. Crack the eggs then place in a mixing bowl.

2. Add softened cream cheese to the bowl then using an electric mixer whisk until smooth and fluffy.

3. Add almond yogurt and cinnamon to the batter then mix well.

4. Preheat a pan over medium heat then coat the pan with cooking spray.

5. Drop about two tablespoons of batter then make the pancake. Repeat with the remaining ingredients.

6. Arrange the pancakes on a serving dish then serve immediately.

NUTRITION PER SERVING

CALORIES 248 PROTEIN 13.8 FIBER 0.8 SUGARS 1 FAT 20.1

TIP

If you like fresh fruit, you can add diced fresh strawberry or blueberry to the batter.

QUICK TOMATO FRITTATA

SERVES 4 PREPARATION TIME 10 MINUTES
COOKING TIME 15 MINUTES

INGREDIENTS
10 organic eggs
1 cup chopped onion
¾ cup crumbled feta cheese
1 cup cherry tomatoes
1 tbsp. butter
2 tbsp. chopped parsley
¼ tsp. salt
½ tsp. black pepper

INSTRUCTIONS

1. Preheat oven to 200°F.

2. Crack the eggs then season with salt and pepper. Whisk until incorporated.

3. Preheat a pan over medium heat then add butter to the pan.

4. Once the butter is melted, stir in chopped onion then sauté until aromatic. Remove from heat.

5. Pour the eggs into the pan then spread evenly.

6. Top the frittata with crumbled feta cheese and halved cherry tomatoes then bake for approximately 10 minutes or until the frittata is set.

7. Remove from heat and let it cool.

8. Serve and enjoy.

NUTRITION PER SERVING

CALORIES 278 PROTEIN 18.7 FIBER 1.3 SUGARS 4.4 FAT 20

TIP

Add some other ingredients that you like to this frittata. Mushrooms, sausage, ground beef, or vegetables are all great choices.

CREAMY ASPARAGUS QUICHE

SERVES 4 PREPARATION TIME 15 MINUTES
COOKING TIME 60 MINUTES

INGREDIENTS
CRUST:
½ cup almond flour
1 organic egg white
1 tbsp. butter
FILLING:
3 organic eggs
1 organic egg yolk
2 tbsp. cooked ground beef
½ cup almond milk
2 tbsp. grated cheese
½ cup chopped asparagus
¼ tsp. salt
¼ tsp. pepper
¼ tsp. nutmeg

INSTRUCTIONS

1. Preheat oven to 375°F then coat a medium pie pan with cooking spray.

2. Combine almond flour with egg white and butter then mix until it becomes a sticky dough.

3. Put the dough into the prepared pie pan then press on the bottom and up the side of the pan.

4. Bake the crust for about 10 minutes then take it out of the oven. Set aside.

5. Crack the eggs then place in a bowl. Season with salt, nutmeg, and pepper.

6. Add egg yolk to the bowl then whisk all until fluffy.

7. Pour almond milk into the eggs then stir well.

8. Sprinkle ground beef and asparagus over the crust then pour in the egg and almond milk mixture.

9. Sprinkle grated cheese on top then bake for about 30 minutes.

10. Once it is done, remove from the oven then place on a cooling rack.

11. Take the quiche out of the pan then cut into wedges.

12. Serve and enjoy.

NUTRITION PER SERVING

CALORIES 308 PROTEIN 19.6 FIBER 1.5 SUGARS 1.8 FAT 24.4

TIP

Do not over bake the quiche to keep the filling soft and to avoid the crust burning. Once the filling is set, remove from the oven.

BEEF AND CAULIFLOWER IN PAN WITH AVOCADO

SERVES 4 PREPARATION TIME 10 MINUTES
COOKING TIME 30 MINUTES

INGREDIENTS
2 tbsp. butter
1 cup chopped onion
1 cup ground beef
¼ tsp. salt
½ tsp. black pepper
1 cup cauliflower florets
5 organic eggs
1 ripe avocado

INSTRUCTIONS

1. Preheat oven to 250°F then coat a casserole dish with cooking spray. Set aside.

2. Preheat a skillet over medium heat then add butter to the skillet.

3. Once the butter is melted, stir in chopped onion then sauté until wilted and aromatic.

6. Pour water over the chicken then cook until the water is completely absorbed.

7. Add green beans and firm egg whites to the skillet then stir well.

8. Transfer to a serving dish then enjoy.

NUTRITION PER SERVING

CALORIES 204 PROTEIN 27.5 FIBER 2.9 SUGARS 1.8 FAT 6.8

CHEESY STUFFED TOMATOES

SERVES 4 PREPARATION TIME 10 MINUTES
COOKING TIME 12 MINUTES

INGREDIENTS
8 red tomatoes
1 cup grated mozzarella cheese
1 tbsp. chopped onion
½ tsp. black pepper

INSTRUCTIONS

1. Preheat oven to 200°F then line a baking sheet with parchment paper.

2. Cut the tomatoes on top, hollow out, then fill each tomato with chopped onion.

3. Top each tomato with grated Mozzarella cheese then sprinkle black pepper over the cheese.

4. Arrange the filled tomatoes on the prepared baking pan then bake for about 10 minutes or until the Mozzarella cheese is melted.

5. Transfer to a serving dish.

6. Enjoy.

NUTRITION PER SERVING

CALORIES 55 PROTEIN 3.7 FIBER 2.3 SUGARS 4.9
FAT 1.6

TIP

Choose ripe tomatoes with firm textures.
To ensure freshness, buy organic tomatoes from
the nearest local market or supermarket.

VERY BERRY SMOOTHIE

SERVES 4 PREPARATION TIME 4 MINUTES
COOKING TIME 6 MINUTES

INGREDIENTS

1 1/2 cups unsweetened almond milk
1 cup chopped strawberries
½ cup blueberries
½ cup raspberries
2 tbsp. lemon juice

INSTRUCTIONS

1. Place strawberries, raspberries, and blueberries in a blender then splash lemon juice over the berries.

2. Pour almond milk into the blender then blend until smooth.

3. Divide the smoothies into 4 serving glasses then serve.

4. Enjoy.

NUTRITION PER SERVING

CALORIES 42 PROTEIN 0.9 FIBER 2.4 SUGARS 4.4

FAT 1.2

TIP

To enhance the freshness sensation of this smoothie, freeze the blueberries, raspberries, and strawberries the night before.

VEGETABLE CHEESE MUFFINS

SERVES 4 PREPARATION TIME 10 MINUTES
COOKING TIME 30 MINUTES

INGREDIENTS
1-1/2 tsp. butter
¾ cup broccoli florets
1-½ cups almond flour
2 organic eggs
¾ cup unsweetened almond milk

INSTRUCTIONS

1. Preheat oven to 200°F then coat 8 muffin cups with cooking spray. Set aside.

2. Crack the eggs then separate the yolk and the egg whites.

3. Using a hand mixer whisk the egg whites until fluffy then set aside.

4. In a separate bowl, combine egg yolk with almond milk and flour then stir well.

5. Melt butter then add to the almond and egg mixture.

6. Stir in egg whites then mix until incorporated.

7. Put broccoli florets in the prepared muffin cups then pour batter to cover.

8. Bake the muffins for about 30 minutes or until a toothpick inserted comes out clean.

9. Remove from the oven then place on a cooling rack.

10. Serve and enjoy.

NUTRITION PER SERVING

CALORIES 213 PROTEIN 9.5 FIBER 3.6 SUGARS 1.5 FAT 17.9

CREAMY BAKED EGGS

SERVES 4 PREPARATION TIME 8 MINUTES
COOKING TIME 32 MINUTES

INGREDIENTS
4 organic eggs
½ cup cherry tomatoes
1 ½ tbsp. coconut oil
½ cup chopped onion
1 tsp. minced garlic
¼ tsp. pepper
1 cup chopped spinach
¼ cup coconut milk

INSTRUCTIONS

1. First, make the creamy spinach.

2. Preheat a medium skillet over medium heat then stir in chopped onion and minced garlic. Sauté until wilted and aromatic.

3. Add chopped spinach to the skillet then cook until just wilted but still bright green.

4. Pour coconut milk over the spinach then season with pepper. Bring to a simmer. Remove from heat.

5. Coat 4 small round baking pans with coconut oil.

6. Divide the cooked spinach into the 4 prepared baking pans then drop an egg in each baking pan.

7. Cut the cherry tomatoes into halves then sprinkle on top.

8. Preheat oven to 250°F then bake the eggs.

9. Once the white eggs are set, remove from the oven then place on a cooling rack.

10. Serve and enjoy.

NUTRITION PER SERVING

CALORIES 154 PROTEIN 6.5 FIBER 1.1 SUGARS 2.1 FAT 13.1

TIP

This dish will taste best if the egg yolk is not overcooked. However, if you don't like a half-cooked egg, you can add cooking time until it is cooked to your liking.

LUNCH

AVOCADO TUNA SALAD

SERVES 4 PREPARATION TIME 5 MINUTES
COOKING TIME 10 MINUTES

INGREDIENTS
**4 ripe avocados
¼ tsp. pepper
2 tbsp. butter
2 tbsp. lemon juice
1 tbsp. chopped parsley**

INSTRUCTIONS

1. Peel the avocados and discard the pits.

2. Cut the avocados into cubes then set aside.

3. Splash lemon juice over the tuna then let it sit for about 2 minutes.

4. Next, preheat a skillet then add butter to the skillet.

5. Once the butter is melted, stir in tuna chunks then season with pepper.

6. Using a wooden spatula, stir the tuna until completely cooked then add avocado cubes to the skillet. Stir until just combined then remove from heat.

7. Transfer to a serving dish then sprinkle chopped parsley on top.

8. Serve and enjoy.

NUTRITION PER SERVING

CALORIES 131 PROTEIN 6.2 FIBER 3.1 SUGARS 0.2 FAT 11.1

TIP

Besides tuna, you can also use salmon, and shrimp for this recipe.
For a healthy twist can add vegetables to this dish.

SAVORY SAUTEED MUSHROOMS

SERVES 4 PREPARATION TIME 5 MINUTES
COOKING TIME 10 MINUTES

INGREDIENTS

4 cups chopped mushrooms
2 tsp. olive oil
3 tsp. minced garlic
½ tsp. black pepper
2 tsp. red chilli flakes
1 tbsp. sesame seeds
¼ cup chopped tomato
1 cup low sodium chicken broth

INSTRUCTIONS

1. Preheat a skillet over medium heat then pour olive oil into the skillet.

2. Stir in minced garlic then sauté until lightly golden and aromatic.

3. Add chopped mushrooms to the skillet then season with pepper and chilli flakes.

4. Pour low sodium chicken broth over the mushrooms then cook until the broth reduces by half.

5. Stir in chopped tomato then mix well.

6. Transfer to a serving dish then sprinkle sesame seeds on top.

7. Serve and enjoy.

NUTRITION PER SERVING

CALORIES 58 PROTEIN 3.4 FIBER 1.3 SUGARS 1.6 FAT 3.7

TIP

You can try various mushrooms for this recipe. White mushrooms, oyster mushrooms, Portobello, and shiitake are all good in this recipe.

EGGS IN A CAVE

SERVES 4 PREPARATION TIME 15 MINUTES
COOKING TIME 25 MINUTES

INGREDIENTS
4 boiled eggs
1 organic egg
2 cups ground beef
¼ tsp. salt
½ tsp. pepper
½ tsp. nutmeg
2 tbsp. coconut flour

INSTRUCTIONS

1. Peel the boiled eggs then set aside.

2. Preheat a steamer over medium heat.

3. Season the beef with salt, pepper, and nutmeg then mix well.

4. Add egg and coconut flour to the beef mixture then stir to combine.

5. Cover each boiled egg with beef mixture then wrap each in aluminium foil.

6. Place the wrapped eggs in the steamer then steam for about 25 minutes.

7. Take the wrapped eggs out of the steamer then let them cool.

8. When the eggs are cool, unwrap the eggs then cut into halves.

9. Arrange on a serving dish then serve.

10. Enjoy.

NUTRITION PER SERVING

CALORIES 225 PROTEIN 20.5 FIBER 1.4 SUGARS 0.8 FAT 14.3

TIP

You can substitute the beef with chicken, lamb, or fish, as you desire. However, you must add more flour to the mixture because those kinds of meat are less firm than beef.
For a smaller size, use boiled quail eggs for the filling.

MIXED VEGETABLES IN TURMERIC GRAVY

SERVES 4 PREPARATION TIME 8 MINUTES
COOKING TIME 18 MINUTES

INGREDIENTS

1 cup chopped cabbage
½ cup chopped carrot
½ cup chopped green beans
1 tsp. sliced garlic
2 tsp. sliced shallot
½ tsp. coriander
½ tsp. pepper
½ tsp. turmeric
1 lemon grass
1 bay leaf
1 tsp. olive oil
1 cup water
1 cup coconut milk

INSTRUCTIONS

1. Preheat a medium skillet then pour olive oil into the skillet.

2. Stir in sliced garlic and shallot then sauté until brown and aromatic.

3. Add cabbage, carrot, and green beans to the skillet then sauté until wilted.

4. Season the vegetables with coriander; pepper, turmeric, lemon grass, and bay leaf then pour water over the vegetables. Bring to boil.

5. Once it is boiling, pour coconut milk into the skillet then bring to a simmer.

6. Transfer to a serving dish then enjoy warm.

NUTRITION PER SERVING

CALORIES 168 PROTEIN 2.1 FIBER 2.8 SUGARS 3.5 FAT 15.6

CHICKEN MEATBALLS IN TOMATO SAUCE

SERVES 4 PREPARATION TIME 14 MINUTES
COOKING TIME 25 MINUTES

INGREDIENTS
1 lb. ground chicken
2 organic eggs
4 cloves garlic
SAUCE:
1 cup diced tomato
½ cup tomato puree
½ cup low sodium chicken broth
¼ tsp. salt
½ tsp. pepper
½ tsp. nutmeg

INSTRUCTIONS

1. Pour about a quart of water into a pot then bring to boil.

2. Meanwhile, combine ground chicken with eggs and garlic then mix well.

3. Shape the mixture into small balls then set aside.

4. Once the water is boiled, stir in the meatballs and cook until the meatballs are floating.

5. While waiting for the meatballs, pour diced tomato, tomato puree, and chicken broth in a saucepan.

6. Season with salt, pepper, and nutmeg then bring to a simmer.

7. Stir occasionally then remove from heat. Set aside.

8. Once the meatballs are floating, strain the meatballs and place on a serving dish.

9. Drizzle the tomato sauce over the meatballs then serve.

10. Enjoy.

NUTRITION PER SERVING

CALORIES 275 PROTEIN 37 FIBER 1.3 SUGARS 3
FAT 10.9

DELICIOUS SALMON ROLL

SERVES 4 PREPARATION TIME 8 MINUTES
COOKING TIME 17 MINUTES

INGREDIENTS
1 lb. salmon fillet
½ cup chopped onion
1 tsp. pepper
2 tbsp. olive oil
2 tbsp. red chilli flakes
1 lb. fresh cabbage

INSTRUCTIONS

1. Preheat a skillet on stove then add butter to the skillet.

2. Once the butter is hot, stir in chopped onion then sauté until wilted and aromatic.

3. Shred the salmon then add to the skillet.

4. Cook until the salmon is no longer pink then add pepper and red chilli flakes. Remove from heat.

5. Steam the cabbage until wilted then place on a flat surface.

6. Top each steamed cabbage with cooked salmon then tightly roll the cabbage.

7. Place the rolled cabbage on a serving dish then enjoy.

NUTRITION PER SERVING

CALORIES 246 PROTEIN 23.7 FIBER 3.4 SUGARS 4.3 FAT 14.2

TIP
Always choose fresh cabbage with wide leaves. This will help you roll the cabbage easier.

BEEF AND CHEESE LASAGNE

SERVES 4 PREPARATION TIME 8 MINUTES
COOKING TIME 36 MINUTES

INGREDIENTS

**2 cups ground beef
1 cup chopped onion
1 tsp. pepper
½ cup low sodium beef broth
½ cup grated cheese
1 cup almond flour
2 organic eggs**

INSTRUCTIONS

1. Combine ground beef with chopped onion and pepper then set aside.

2. Place almond flour in a mixing bowl then add organic eggs.

3. Pour beef broth over the almond flour mixture, using an electric mixer to whisk until incorporated.

4. Preheat a pan over medium heat then coat with cooking spray.

5. Make thin omelettes with the almond mixture then set aside.

6. Coat a casserole dish with cooking spray then place an omelette on the bottom.

7. Layer with the beef mixture then repeat with the remaining beef and omelettes.

8. Sprinkle grated cheese on top then set aside.

9. Preheat oven to 300°F then bake the lasagne for about 30 minutes or until the cheese is lightly golden.

10. Once it is done, remove from the oven then let it cool for a few minutes.

11. Serve and enjoy.

NUTRITION PER SERVING

CALORIES 266 PROTEIN 19.3 FIBER 1.5 SUGARS
1.8 FAT 19.1

TIP

If you want a brighter taste, you can drizzle tomato
puree between every layer of the lasagne.

SPICY CHICKEN STEW

SERVES 4 PREPARATION TIME 8 MINUTES
COOKING TIME 22 MINUTES

INGREDIENTS
1.5 lbs. chicken wings
3 cloves garlic
5 shallots
3 candlenuts
1 inch galangal
1 bay leaf
¼ cup red chilli
2 kefir lime leaves
1 lemon grass
3 cups low sodium chicken broth

INSTRUCTIONS

1. Place garlic, shallots, candlenuts, and red chillies in a food processor. Pulse until combined.

2. Transfer the spice mixture to a skillet then add galangal, bay leaf, lime leaf, and lemon grass to the skillet.

3. Arrange the chicken wings over the spices then pour chicken broth over the chicken wings. Bring to boil.

4. Once it is boiling, reduce the heat then cook until the chicken broth has reduced to approximately one cup.

5. Transfer the spicy chicken stew to a serving dish then serve warm.

NUTRITION PER SERVING

CALORIES 138 PROTEIN 6 FIBER 2.1 SUGARS 1.1
FAT 8.9

SMOOTH PUMPKIN SOUP

SERVES 4 PREPARATION TIME 8 MINUTES
COOKING TIME 25 MINUTES

INGREDIENTS
3 cups pumpkin cubes
½ tsp. black pepper
1 ½ cup coconut milk
2 tbsp. chopped parsley

INSTRUCTIONS

1. Place the pumpkin in a steamer then steam until tender.

2. Transfer the steamed pumpkin to a blender then pour coconut milk into the blender.

3. Season with black pepper then blend until smooth.

4. Pour the smooth pumpkin into a saucepan then bring to a simmer.

5. Transfer to a serving bowl then serve warm.

NUTRITION PER SERVING

CALORIES 71 PROTEIN 1 FIBER 1 SUGARS 1.2 FAT 5.4

CRISPY CABBAGE SALAD

SERVES 4 PREPARATION TIME 8 MINUTES
COOKING TIME 5 MINUTES

INGREDIENTS
1 lb. cabbage
3 tbsp. mayonnaise
¼ cup almond yogurt
3 tbsp. lemon juice

INSTRUCTIONS

1. Shred the cabbage then place in a salad bowl.

2. Drizzle mayonnaise and almond yogurt over the cabbage then splash lemon juice on top. Toss to combine.

3. Cover the salad with a lid then refrigerate for a minimum of 2 hours.

4. Remove from the refrigerator then enjoy cold.

NUTRITION PER SERVING

CALORIES 85 PROTEIN 1.9 FIBER 3 SUGARS 5.2

FAT 4.4

TIP
To enhance the health content, you can add shredded carrot or cucumber to this salad.

ASPARAGUS TUNA PIE

SERVES 4 PREPARATION TIME 4 MINUTES
COOKING TIME 32 MINUTES

INGREDIENTS
2 tsp. butter
¼ cup chopped onion
1 cup chopped asparagus
¼ cup green peas
½ cup tuna chunks
4 organic eggs
½ tsp. pepper

INSTRUCTIONS

1. Preheat oven to 250°F then coat a casserole dish with cooking spray.

2. Sprinkle chopped onion on the bottom of the prepared dish then layer with asparagus, peas, and tuna chunks.

3. Crack the eggs then season with pepper. Mix until incorporated.

4. Pour the beaten eggs over the tuna then drop pieces of butter on top.

5. Bake for about 30 minutes until the eggs are set.

6. Remove from the oven then let cool for a few minutes.

7. Once you want to enjoy, cut the pie into wedges then serve.

NUTRITION PER SERVING

CALORIES 109 PROTEIN 9.4 FIBER 1.4 SUGARS 1.8 FAT 6.5

TIP

This dish can be prepared in advance. Cover the top with plastic wrap then microwave whenever you want to consume.

BAKED CHICKEN NUGGETS

SERVES 4 PREPARATION TIME 10 MINUTES
COOKING TIME 20 MINUTES

INGREDIENTS

**2 lbs. ground chicken
2 tsp. minced garlic
½ tsp. pepper
3 organic eggs
½ cup coconut flour
2 tbsp. coconut milk**

INSTRUCTIONS

1. Place ground chicken in a food processor then add minced garlic, pepper, and 2 tablespoons of coconut flour. Pulse to combine.

2. Crack the eggs then place in a bowl.

3. Pour coconut milk into the eggs then mix well.

4. Add the egg mixture to the chicken mixture then stir until incorporated.

5. Shape the chicken nuggets into medium cubes then roll in the remaining coconut flour.

6. Preheat oven to 300°F then line a baking sheet with parchment paper.

7. Arrange the chicken cubes on the prepared baking sheet then bake for about 20 minutes or until the chicken cubes are lightly golden.

8. Remove from the oven then transfer to a serving dish.

9. Serve and enjoy.

NUTRITION PER SERVING

CALORIES 235 PROTEIN 24.2 FIBER 0.9 SUGARS 0.6 FAT 14.4

TIP

Some people love to add vegetables to these nuggets. For sure, it is the best way to make children eat their vegetables.

Conclusion

As you have seen, the keto diet requires a bit of careful planning and preparation. But once you've started, you'll begin to see what all the fuss is about. Taking care to count the net carbs in everything you eat will soon pay off and you'll see the pounds dropping off, every time you stand on the scales, or look in the mirror.

Don't feel disheartened if you feel a little unwell at the beginning of your journey, or if you hit a plateau later on in your journey and the weight seems slow to drop off. There are ups and downs to everyone's journey and at the beginning, when your body is still adjusting to ketosis, it's usual to feel a little off.

As long as you are careful to track your grams of net carbs accurately, you can be sure that you'll maintain ketosis, and you'll begin to feel lighter, healthier and even have more energy and focus than ever before. Join the plethora of people who have found success and happiness in their lives through following the keto diet. Today is the day that you can make a change!

Useful References

www.webmd.com
www.start.perfectketo.com
www.dietdoctor.com
www.healthline.com
www.thrivestrive.com
www.rebootedbody.com
www.medicalnewstoday.com
www.ruled.me
www.myketocoach.com
www.ketodietapp.com
www.lowcarbediem.com

All information is intended only to help you cooperate with your doctor, in your efforts toward desirable weight levels and health. Only your doctor can determine what is right for you. In addition to regular check ups and medical supervision, from your doctor, before starting any other weight loss program, you should consult with your personal physician.

FN№

Presented by French Number Publishing
French Number Publishing is an independent
publishing house headquartered in Paris, France
with offices in North America, Europe, and Asia.
FN№ is committed to connect the most promising
writers to readers from all around the world.
Together we aim to explore the most challenging
issues on a large variety of topics that are of
interest to the modern society.

FN№